Managing Intimacy and Emotions in Advanced Fertility Care

Other Health & Social Care books from M&K include:

Inter-professional Approaches to Young Fathers
ISBN: 978-1-905539-29-1 · 2008

Pre-Teen and Teenage Pregnancy:
A 21st century reality
ISBN: 978-1-905539-11-6 · 2007

Research Issues in Health and Social Care
ISBN: 978-1-905539-20-8 · 2009

Nurses and Their Patients:
Informing practice through psychodynamic insights
ISBN: 978-1-905539-31-4 · 2009

Improving Patient Outcomes:
A resource for ward leaders
ISBN: 978-1-905539-06-2 · 2007

Perspectives on Death and Dying
ISBN: 978-1-905539-21-5 · 2009

Identification and Treatment of Alcohol Dependency
ISBN: 978-1-905539-16-1 · 2009

Nutrition for Children:
A no nonsense guide for parents
ISBN: 978-1-905539-26-0 · 2008

Routine Blood Results Explained
ISBN: 978-1-905539-38-3 · 2007

Deep Vein Thrombosis and Pulmonary Embolism:
A guide for practitioners
ISBN: 978-1-905539-51-2 · 2009

Managing Intimacy and Emotions in Advanced Fertility Care

The future of nursing and midwifery roles

Helen Therese Allan

Managing Intimacy and Emotions in Advanced Fertility Care:
The future of nursing and midwifery roles
Helen Allan

ISBN: 978-1-905539-07-9

First published 2009

British Library Cataloguing in Publication Data
A catalogue record for this book is available from the British Library

Notice
Clinical practice and medical knowledge constantly evolve. Standard safety precautions must be followed, but, as knowledge is broadened by research, changes in practice, treatment and drug therapy may become necessary or appropriate. Readers must check the most current product information provided by the manufacturer of each drug to be administered and verify the dosages and correct administration, as well as contraindications. It is the responsibility of the practitioner, utilising the experience and knowledge of the patient, to determine dosages and the best treatment for each individual patient. Any brands mentioned in this book are as examples only and are not endorsed by the Publisher. Neither the Publisher nor the authors assume any liability for any injury and/or damage to persons or property arising from this publication.

The Publisher
To contact M&K Publishing write to:
M&K Update Ltd · The Old Bakery · St. John's Street
Keswick · Cumbria CA12 5AS
Tel: 01768 773030 · Fax: 01768 781099
publishing@mkupdate.co.uk
www.mkupdate.co.uk

Designed and typeset in 11pt Usherwood Book by Mary Blood
Printed in England

Contents

Acknowledgements are due to the staff and patients of
the two assisted reproduction clinics in which I have gathered
data; to fertility nurses and counsellors with whom I have had
conversations over the years and to those anonymous referees
who gave their thoughtful comments on the papers upon
which this book is based.

Chapter 1
Introduction

There are a number of books which focus on emotions in specific areas of health care practice. Many of these focus on working with emotions in mental health, psychology and cognitive behaviour therapy. There are far fewer which deal with the role of emotions and how to work with emotions in nursing and midwifery (Griffiths 1998; Katz 2006) although a recent edited book by Hunter & Deery (forthcoming) has dealt with emotions in midwifery practice. A number of general textbooks deal with emotions in therapy and can be applied to nursing (Frost 2003; Turner 2007; Robertson & Freshwater 2002). Of these, three focus on working with emotions and sexuality (Wells 2000; Irwin 2002; Savage 2003) which is, of course, central to assisted reproduction[1] nursing and the experience of infertility. Wells and Irwin are nurses trained in psychosexual nursing practice and members of the Association of Psychosexual Nursing. The association trains nurses in Balint seminars to work with psychosexual issues brought to the nurse–patient consultation. It aims to 'recognise and respond constructively to the psychosexual issues encountered in their everyday practice' (Irwin 2006:445). Savage's report is a study of this Balint seminar training approach.

I was introduced to the work of the Association of Psychosexual Nursing by Marjorie Rutter who was a counsellor in the assisted reproduction (AR) unit at Kings College Hospital until she retired. She and I developed a module for nurses studying for their Diploma in Fertility Nursing accredited by the Royal College of Nursing. The module was called 'The Helping Relationship' and was a way of training fertility nurses to work with emotions – their own and their patients. The assumptions underpinning this

---

[1] I shall call nursing in assisted reproduction clinics assisted reproduction nursing rather than fertility nursing as AR clinics are increasingly becoming known as assisted reproduction clinics and the term is more widely used internationally.

module (and this book) are that if nursing is about working with rather than doing things to people, and relating to people as partners in their care, the nurse is likely to become emotionally engaged with the people she meets in her professional work. Working with people experiencing difficulties relating to their fertility and their ability to conceive, can be exciting, challenging, rewarding and fulfilling. It can also be demanding and anxiety provoking. It is the emotional nature of the work that this module sought to support through focusing and reflecting on the nurse–patient relationship and what occurs within this. The nurses who undertook this module explored how they worked with infertile people and developed skills and confidence relating to the psychosexual and emotional side of assisted conception. Their skills included inquiring about emotional and sexual matters with patients and being able to respond to pain and distress which may be expressed overtly or covertly during the consultation.

It was an experiential and participative module and was emotionally challenging or difficult at times as students reflected on their own feelings, thoughts and behaviours within the nurse–patient relationship.

This book arises from my experiences as an infertility patient as well as my experiences in research and teaching in this field, in particular from awareness that managing emotions is difficult for nurses and any health professional in this area. My awareness was stimulated at first by the findings in study 1 and then by working with students and Marjorie Rutter on the Helping Relationship module; through attending to their own and their patients' emotions, in a supportive and learning environment, they were able to change their practice and support patients more effectively. A purpose of this book is to focus on an unexplored area of fertility or AR nursing practice, namely working with emotions, and to promote awareness of how emotions affect the nurse and the patient dynamic in AR clinics and in women's health more widely in the context of nursing role developments.

An historical look at managing emotions in AR nursing

An historical look

Taylor (personal communication) argues that the emotional toil of caring for people in sickness and as they die is rarely referred to in policy, yet stress is, of course, inevitable when working with sick patients and their relatives (Katz 2006; Frost 2003). And indeed what is lacking in the nursing and midwifery literature – besides a consideration of the psychological, socio-economic and politico-structural factors which influence infertility services more generally, and fertility nursing in particular – is an in-depth exploration of the psychological and emotional consequences of infertility for infertile people. It is the experience of emotions for infertile patients and staff caring for them, and how these emotions are managed by patients and staff, which formed the main findings from study 1.

Fineman (2004) argues that descriptions of organisations are often bland and do not paint a picture of the emotional component of working life. He suggests that the study of emotions at work allows two processes to emerge. Firstly, people, their behaviours and the effects of those behaviours come to the fore and become the focus of study. Secondly, emotions are understood to be the main medium through which people act and interact. The ignoring of emotions between staff as a result of work relationships is what Frost (2003) refers to as 'toxic' emotions, where emotions are ignored and become harmful to creativity in organisations. However, I wish to focus in this book on the emotions which arise as a result of caring for infertile people as they enter into AR clinics and become patients rather than the emotions which arise from staff relationships (although these are of course crucial to how organisations function [Menzies 1971]).

In my research, through observations in two AR clinics, it was clear that the organisation of nursing work was anything but bland. Indeed, it seemed to me that the organisation of nursing work and the clinics was shaped by the anxiety raised by emotions evoked by the experience of being infertile on the one hand and caring for infertile people on the other. The clinics were organised into public and private spaces ensuring that the potentially disruptive emotions of staff and patients were controlled and largely unexpressed or if expressed to, unacknowledged by, the staff.

Managing intimacy and emotions

The findings demonstrated that the expression of caring behaviours by staff depended on the use of space within the clinic and that the nurses, working mostly in the public spaces of the clinic, used these public spaces to distance themselves from patients' emotions. I did not see this distanced caring as a negative aspect of nursing; I argued that this distance was necessary to help the nurses defend against the anxiety evoked through caring for infertile patients. It was simply very hard emotional work which was unsupported.

My first piece of postdoctoral work, in collaboration with Debbie Barber, an AR nurse specialist, explored issues of intimacy and nurse–patient relationships further. We used Menzies' insight that nurse–patient relationships change 'ordinary' social relationships and that there is a need to manage the intimate and emotional nature of these clinical, 'non-social' relationships (Menzies 1970). We argued that advanced roles offered ways of managing intimacy positively for patients and nurses because these roles allowed continuity of care – patients saw 'their' nurse more frequently and this allowed them to feel safe. These relationships were not however intimate in the sense that each side knew each other well; the nurse–patient relationship continued to be distanced rather than intimate. Definitions of intimacy in the nursing literature suggest that intimacy is the opportunity provided in 'the basic work of nursing [...] for a psychological closeness or meaningful relationship between nurse and patient that may hold therapeutic potential' (Savage 1995:11). Our findings suggested that 'distanced' nurse–patient relationships which developed in advanced nursing roles were positive because they helped nurses and patients manage their emotions during difficult and intrusive intimate examinations while at the same time allowing continuity for nurse and patient.

Advanced AR roles included nurses undertaking tasks which were formerly performed by doctors. Rather than limiting the potential for intimacy between the nurse and the fertility patient, we argue that such roles allow the nurse to provide increased continuity of care. This continuity of care facilitates the management of emotions where a feeling of closeness is created while at the same time maintaining a distance or safe boundary which both nurses and patients are comfortable with.

More recently, I've developed an interest in technologies and emotions after a study trip to Australia and New Zealand funded by the Florence Nightingale Foundation. The expansion and consequent changes in the delivery of care to couples seeking in vitro fertilisation (IVF) in Australia and New Zealand have led to:

- an increased number of cycles per clinic
- the organisation of clinic work as telecare, i.e. nurses maintain relationships with patients via the use of email and telephones
- the increasing management of patients at a distance, i.e. the patient attends the main clinic perhaps once for the initial consultation and then for the egg collection, embryo transfer and otherwise attends a satellite clinic
- a return to task allocation for nurses.

These developments in Australia and New Zealand raise questions about how nurses manage emotions and develop meaningful relationships with patients who are now managed at a distance from the AR clinics. And they pose some questions about the future of advanced fertility roles in the UK if such developments occur here.

This book is based on papers from empirical research I have written over a period of 10 years; two of the papers were written in collaboration with Debbie Barber who works at the Radcliffe Fertility Unit in Oxford in the UK. The book seeks to discuss the implications of the role developments in fertility nursing as well as address the challenges that an expanding assisted reproductive technology market holds for maintaining therapeutic, caring relationships with nurses. While this book considers AR nursing in particular, the arguments I make about the management of intimacy and emotions apply to nursing more generally and women's health and midwifery more specifically, largely because role development, the nature of caring and the management of emotions are issues which affect all areas of nursing practice (see among others, Allen 2004). In addition, the gendered nature of AR nursing, which is a significant feature of the data, makes the findings applicable to gynaecology nursing which is also strongly gendered (Bolton 2005). Therefore, the findings presented in Chapters 2 to 5 could be applied to any setting in women's health including midwifery; while the findings presented in Chapters 7 to 8 could be applied to any nursing setting.

Managing intimacy and emotions

The aim of the book

The aim of this book is to consider the nature of advanced AR nursing roles in the 21st century in three contexts:

1. The rapidly expanding provision of assisted reproductive technologies (ARTs) which are increasingly successful. In the UK, while the rate of couples undergoing in vitro fertilisation (IVF) remained relatively stable during the 1990s, the success rate of IVF has risen and the risks fallen (HFEA, 2005/2006). The number of couples in the UK experiencing fertility problems has risen, with 1.4% of all births in the UK as the result of infertility treatments (HFEA, 2005/2006).

2. The changes and developments of nursing roles in general, and AR nursing roles in particular. These changes and developments have been driven by policy such as the United Kingdom Central Council's (UKCC) Higher Level of Practice Project (2002), the UKCC's Scope of Professional Practice (1992), the Future of Professional Regulation (UKCC 1998) and the reduction in junior doctors' hours (DH 2003).

3. Awareness that emotions and emotional care are important components of health care delivery. Nurses have continued to work in Balint seminar groups to explore the 'psychodynamics of the doctor/nurse–patient relationship' (Savage 2003:10). And more recently, in nursing, a focus on the therapeutic potential of the nurse–patient relationship achieved through reflection and supervision has been prominent in both academic and practice literature (Savage 1995; Wilkins *et al.* 1997). However, while emotions in nursing have been explored in terms of gender and the management of feelings (Davies 1995; James 1992; Smith 1992) there has been very little 'practical' discussion of how these approaches can be used in nursing generally. Neither has AR nursing addressed the emotional side of its work in consistent publications, education or training.

Who is this book for?

This book is intended for nurses and midwives who work in AR clinics and those who either work in, or have an interest in women's health. As has been stated, the number of IVF births is increasing steadily as a percentage of all births and therefore infertility may be said to be increasingly influential in women's health nursing and midwifery. I am constantly impressed by the sense of connectedness which women caring for women express and as the data in this book shows, women patients feel that there is something special about being cared for by female nurses and midwives. The emotions raised in clinical practice for nurses and midwives caring for women need attention and discussion and this book is intended to contribute to a greater awareness of emotions in clinical practice even in a busy NHS. Indeed, paying attention to emotions when you are busy may help you understand and deal with the business.

This book is intended for practising nurses and midwives and therefore each chapter ends with a reflection from the author on the implications of the data for practice and an opportunity for the reader to reflect on their practice too.

The British context of infertility

The British context of infertility

In the UK, investigations of infertility are undertaken by couples' general practitioners (GPs) in primary care and as such are provided by the National Health Service (NHS); the NHS is a publicly funded health service. And the provision of services is governed by the guidelines from NICE (National Institute for Health and Clinical Excellence) which advises the NHS about whether or not treatments and investigations are clinically and cost effective for use in the NHS. The NICE guideline for infertility (2004) (www.nice.org.uk/Guidance/CG11) recommends that suitable couples should receive up to three IVF cycles on the NHS, that is, free of charge if certain conditions are met. These conditions are based on the woman's age (<39 years old) and whether the couple have children by previous relationships; if there are children, no funding is available. However individual primary care trusts (PCTs) who commission secondary care and are restricted by national budgets, continue not to provide NHS treatments. Usually, couples have preliminary investigations with their GP before a referral to an ART clinic. ART clinics are not available in every NHS hospital (or acute NHS Trust) if the PCT does not commission ARTs. Therefore distance may be a factor in accessibility of ARTs especially in rural areas.

Managing intimacy and emotions

In the UK, fertility services are delivered via publicly funded AR clinics and via the private sector. The Human Fertilisation and Embryology Authority (HFEA) in the UK has a legal responsibility to license all units providing assisted reproduction with the use of human gametes, and to consult widely on further policy developments in fertility and embryo research (English 1995; HFEA 2005/6). The nature and availability of infertility treatments have been contentious in the UK as elsewhere (De Lacey 2002). Infertility treatments have not been funded fully and access to any treatments has been described as a 'postcode' lottery (De Lacey 2002; Brinsden 2003). To correct this, the government has allowed the provision of limited NHS funding for infertility treatments (Brinsden 2003). The HFEA (2000) suggests that the prevalence of infertility in the UK population runs at 15%. It is estimated that one in seven couples do not conceive within 1 year of trying for a baby (http://www.nice.org.uk/Guidance/CG11). At the same time as the technological potential to investigate and diagnose infertility has increased, the success rates have remained relatively low despite improvements recently and fertility treatments remain a contested subject (De Lacey 2002).

ARTs are regulated by the national, licensing and regulating authority, the Human Fertilisation and Embryology Authority which has three professional and five lay members. The first Human Fertilisation and Embryology Act was passed in 1990. In 2007, the draft Human Fertilisation and Embryology Bill was presented to parliament for consideration and there has been intense media interest in infertility and the provision of assisted conception. The Bill is important in the context of this book because the provision of counselling services in AR clinics is framed by the HFEA Code of Practice. Significant changes in the new Bill concern the welfare of the child in donor treatments and in treatments for single women.

At present, counselling services are not mandatory under the existing Act except implications counselling for those patients intending to undergo assisted reproduction. Emotional issues are dealt with in clinics in relation to implications counselling rather than counselling in relation to the emotional effects of infertility for patients. In other words, emotions are not at the forefront of the legislation or practice.

The studies themselves

The studies

The data which underpins this book comes from two empirical studies; study 1 was undertaken as a PhD over a period of six years and study 2 as a post-doctoral research project. The second study was a much smaller study. Both studies used an ethnographic case study approach which provides in-depth contextual data to explore people's motivations and behaviours using multiple methods of data collection (Gomm *et al.* 2000). From these case studies, some meaningful analyses of current changes in nursing roles can be made which may then be transferable to other AR units and, possibly, within wider contexts within the NHS (Lincoln & Guba 2000).

Study 1

The aims of this study were to critically analyse the nursing role in two AR clinics in the context of theories of caring and emotions; to voice the meanings that fertility and infertility have for staff and patients and analyse how these shape patient needs and nursing practice; to understand the possible ways in which the structures of the hospital and the outpatient clinic might influence the behaviours of staff.

Method

The setting was a British AR unit, which was spread over two sites for the majority of the period I spent in the field; this effectively meant there were two clinics within the same unit. The two sites were called ACU and BCU. Data was collected over 2 years using participant observation in the clinic and semi-structured interviews with 15 women undergoing infertility treatments and 20 members of staff. Participant observation involved, in total, 48 visits to the clinics of 2 to 3 hours per visit (96 hours minimum) over the same period. Ethical approval was gained through the hospital ethics committee.

This study was conducted in publicly funded or National Health Service AR clinics that offered donor insemination for couples with male factor problems (DI), assisted ovulation for women with polycystic ovarian syndrome, and insemination by husband or partner (AIH) for couples with unexplained infertility. Couples were referred to the AR clinics by their general medical practitioners (GPs) after a period of unprotected sexual intercourse for at least 1 year. Couples seeking in vitro fertilisation (IVF), gamete intrafallopian transfer (GIFT) and intracytoplasmic sperm injection (ICSI) were referred to a private AR clinic in the same building as the NHS AR clinics.

Study 2

The aim of this study was to describe advanced AR nursing roles and to explore the nature of these roles for the nurses undertaking them and for patients being cared for in this new way.

Method

We purposefully selected an AR clinic where these roles were practised as a single case from the small number of AR units where nurses practice in this way. Ethics committee approval was gained from the local research and ethics committee.

Data collection methods included four weeks of participant observation by one of the researchers. Notes from participant observation were analysed by both researchers to identify interview questions for semi-structured interviews with five nurses, one health care assistant, one doctor and three infertile couples.

The data was collected in an AR clinic which offered a full range of investigations and assisted reproductive technologies including IVF, GIFT and ICSI as well as a donor programme. Referrals were from NHS clinics and GPs.

Ethnographic authority

The data in this book presents reflexive accounts of reality built up through the field relationships and developed between the participant observation and interview data. Reflexivity in this instance means acknowledging that the final ethnographic report is not the 'truth'. It is the researcher's representation; indeed, I have shaped and produced it. I am writing this book as a nurse researcher who has been involved with educating and researching fertility nursing for 10 years. However, as will become apparent during the book, I am also infertile and it is this dual position that gives me voice; that is, it is through my personal journey of infertility and motherhood through adoption that I have come to realise the potential of caring through working with emotions in fertility nursing. However this book is written primarily from the voice of the nurse researcher and the patients and staff involved in both these studies.

Presentation of data

In this book, I present anonymised extracts of the interview data verbatim with comments on the themes which emerged in relation to the literature.

The meaning of advanced and specialist nursing roles

It is well established that there are a plethora of titles to describe new nursing roles and that there has been disagreement over their meaning (Daly & Carnwell 2003; Bryant-Lukosius *et al.* 2004). When Debbie Barber and I began study 2, we used the UKCC's (1999a) definition of higher levels of practice to describe the advanced nursing roles we observed nurses performing in practice. Important for us in the UKCC's definition was the idea of 'advanced' meaning 'practitioners using their original knowledge and skills as a basis from which to develop practice'. (UKCC 1999a:1). It also involved for us a sense of specialisation or the provision of care for a specific group of patients with complex health needs (Bryant-Lukosius *et al* 2004:522). However it is clear that other frameworks exist whereby the advanced roles we observed by some AR nurses would be at the level of specialist nurse rather than advanced nurse practitioner or consultant nurse (Daly & Carnwell 2003); the dividing line between levels of practice being the degree to which nurses worked with patients without diagnoses. I have retained the use of the term 'advanced nursing role' in this book allowing for other frameworks because I believe AR nurses who practice in the ways we observed were practicing at an advanced level rather than specialist level.

Structure of the book

Structure of the book

The book is arranged around the assumption that an understanding of emotions and psychoanalytic approaches to reproduction inform nursing practice. There are three sections:

Part I contains the theoretical background to the book:
Chapter 2 presents a brief theoretical overview of caring and emotions. Chapter 3 provides an overview of reproduction and sexuality, and research into the experience of infertility from psychological and psychoanalytic viewpoints.

Part II contains three chapters on caring and the experience of infertility:
Chapter 4 discusses the nature of caring and managing emotions in AR nursing. Chapter 5 presents a discussion of chaperoning and argues that chaperoning, which is considered to be outdated and a waste of skilled nursing time, is actually therapeutic for patients. Chapter 6 focuses on the experience of infertility as a liminal state and suggests that the AR clinic acts to contain the anxiety of this liminal experience while the patient undergoes investigations and treatments.

Part III contains a discussion of contemporary advanced AR nursing:
Chapter 7 focuses on the nature of intimacy and suggests that advanced AR nursing roles provide continuity of care which helps patients and staff manage through emotions evoked through invasive, intimate procedures necessary in assisted reproductive technologies. Chapter 8 considers the nature of advanced AR nursing roles and the reasons nurses undertake them. The data suggests that nurses construct moral narratives to justify taking on advanced roles but these roles are fragile and dependent on both the moral narratives and supportive, collegiate relationships with medical colleagues. Chapter 9 considers the implications of recent developments in assisted reproductive technologies (ARTs) for continuing advanced AR nursing roles and any therapeutic benefit which I have ascribed to them for patients in this book. The discussion then focuses more broadly on women's health to consider the nature of advanced nursing and midwifery practice.

Part I

Theoretical Background

Chapter 2
A theoretical overview of caring and emotions

Caring and emotions influenced the shaping of both the studies upon which this book is based. I start this chapter where I started my PhD in 1993: with myself, my emotions and my responses to care within AR clinics.

There are many definitions of self in the nursing literature (Uys 1980; Forrest 1989; Mahlstedt 1991; Barber 1991). Self, or more specifically, the relationship between the personal and the professional or public self, is central to this book. Years of socialisation as a nurse had taught me that my emotions were private and I should not allow them to intrude on my professional life. My private self was not part of my professional self. I had also learned coping mechanisms to hide my emotional involvement in patients' experiences (Menzies 1970). My generation of nurses was not encouraged to empathise with our patients ... to feel the bonds between us or to experience and vocalise the relationship between patient and self (Uys 1980). Therefore, when I was diagnosed as infertile, at a professional level, I expected little real contact with the nursing staff. Yet, personally, I longed for it; this led to the boundaries between private and professional becoming blurred as my expectations of support as a patient challenged long-held professional beliefs.

At another level, my experience as an infertile woman and a nurse gave me an in-depth understanding of infertility and how the process of investigations and treatments affected patients. I had no opportunity to share this with the nurses I had contact with. But if I did not share this knowledge with the nursing staff, how could they give individualistic care? How could they know my self ... my body, thoughts and sensations? How could they meet my needs? I began to ask how do nurses care if my self (private and professional) was invisible to the nurses. Nurses were on the periphery of my care and I had more contact with the medical than the nursing staff. If the nurses did not care, why were nurses there at all?

At about this time, I decided to leave nursing and go to university. But, ten years later and having resumed my nursing career, it seemed that the central question of the relationship between the private and professional self which was brought into focus by my experiences as an infertile woman and patient, was now being debated within the nursing literature (Barber 1991).

The academic work on caring and intimacy upon which this book is based has developed from my earlier search for a way to be seen and responded to as a patient. This book then explores two broad areas which have developed from my experience. Firstly, the nature of caring in fertility nursing and secondly, the effects that the emotions raised by working in this field have on the care nurses give to their infertile patients.

Understanding caring

Understanding caring

There is a large nursing literature on caring which reflects its presumed importance for nursing. A concern with caring and its relationship to nursing can be seen as far back as Nightingale (1859) and traced through modern nursing theorists such as Peplau (1988). However, it is only in the last 30 years (Leininger 1978; Watson 1988; Benner & Wrubel 1989; Morse *et al* 1990; Swanson 1999) that it has been suggested that caring is central to nursing. And while caring attributes have been identified (e.g. Brilowski & Wendler 2005), others suggest that we are no nearer to defining exactly what caring in nursing is (Paley 2001) or enabling trained nurses to care (Allan 2007b).

Caring is moreover problematic for nursing and nurses (Davies 1995). For example, it is argued that caring and motherhood are associated with women (Chodorow 1989; Sayers 1991) and women's psychology (Harbison 1992; Gilligan 1982; 1993) and caring forms the basis of nursing. This has raised questions about whether women are 'natural' carers (Colliere 1986; Bowden 1997) and therefore 'natural' nurses. This association between women and caring/nursing has led to the devaluing of nursing as an occupation in a patriarchal society where femininity itself is devalued (Davies 1995; Mitchell 1974; Gilligan 1982 and Oakley 1993). However, many women and men would deny that women are either natural carers or indeed the only carers in both western societies and other societies (Oakley 1993).

Another approach to caring is called the ethic of care (Gilligan 1982; Noddings 1984). An ethic of care is an approach to care which is based on the assumption that caring is based on a truthful relationship between carer and cared for which demonstrates concern at all times. The carer deals with each person as an individual. Nursing theorists such as Benner & Wrubel (1989) and Watson (1988) have argued that an ethic of care is at the heart of nursing; Hartman (1998) has argued that nurses have a moral imperative to 'enter into a relationship with clients of nursing' (1998:18). However this approach to care assumes that caring may be undertaken without emotional involvement (Savage 1995; van Schie & Seedhouse 1997) and denies the imbalance of nurse–patient relationships (Kirschenbaum & Henderson 1989). It also underplays the contributions of an ethic of justice as the basis for ethical nursing practice (Kuhse 1997; Brewin 1993) as well as an ethic of care.

These gendered features of caring as the basis of nursing are compounded by the nature of women's work, low pay and exploitative work conditions in health and social care (Thomas 1993; Dalley 1995; Heslop & Oates 1995) in addition to historically, oppressive relationships with medicine (Smith & Agard 1997). Davies (1995) and Porter (1995) (among others) conclude that nursing and caring are low value work within capitalist patriarchal societies. The extent to which nursing is devalued in health care is acknowledged by Oakley (1993:51) who admits that caring and nursing were invisible during 20 years of experience as a social researcher within health care. However, she warns that improving the status of such low value work is a challenge for nurses.

Defining care

Defining care

It is in this context that nursing researchers have tried to define care and assess its contribution to health care. Care has been defined as inherent to the nurse–patient relationship (Travelbee 1971; Uys 1980; Gadow 1985; Ray 1987; Kitson 1987; Meutzal

1988; Ersser 1991; 1997; Hawthorne & Yurkovich 1995; Brilowski & Wendler 2005). Care is seen as a form of therapy and the nurse–patient relationship as therapeutic because the attitude of the carer towards the person cared for is caring and beneficent (Noddings 1984; Reiman 1986; Gadow 1987). Ersser (1997) summarises caring in this tradition as patient centred, involving technical competence to achieve beneficial outcomes and a personal and emotional response to the patient. Ersser's (1997) research into nursing as therapy suggests that nurses utilise their personal qualities and presence to care; they relate to patients in caring and the quality of the nurse's interaction delineates caring. There are specific nursing actions which utilise emotions in an instrumental way, for example, observing a patient's scan while maintaining a conversation.

Secondly, attempts to operationalise and delineate the value of caring have been undertaken (Gardner & Wheeler 1981; 1987; van Essen & Sjoden 1991; Clarke & Wheeler 1992; Forrest 1989; Sanford 2000; Paley 2001). These studies have found that patients expect and want nurses to be kind, sympathetic, comforting and able to communicate as well as competent, have scientific knowledge, technical excellence and skilled efficiency (van Essen & Sjoden 1991; Smith 1992; Clarke & Wheeler 1992; Halldorsdottir & Hamrin 1997; Brilowski & Wendler 2005). However, in contrast to patients' expectations of nurses, nurses expect to have meaningful relationships with patients and emphasise the emotional aspects of their role rather than the efficiency or instrumental aspects (Clarke & Wheeler 1992; Kyle 1995). Integrating the competency and the emotional aspects of caring is brought together in many nursing theories within this tradition. Leininger's theory of nursing is typical (1990). She claims that nursing is the art and science of care/caring and her definition of caring is 'those assistive, supportive or facilitative acts for or towards another individual or group with evident or anticipated needs to ameliorate or improve human condition or lifeways' (Leininger 1990:19).

Lastly, researchers have defined caring in terms of emotion or the emotional connection arising from the nurse–patient relationship. It has been described as 'the public form of private love' (Dunlop 1986:662), 'sentimental work' or TLC (tender loving care) (Strauss et al. 1985) and an emotional phenomenon, love and affection, emotional support (Graham 1993). The idea of emotions arising from caring is also described by Griffin (1983) as energising and motivating. James (1992) and Smith (1992) consider caring may involve an emotional cost if given in public, and use the term care work or emotional labour to emphasise its separation from the private sphere where care is given freely. Smith (1992) and Smith & Agard (1997) consider emotions, feelings, communication and relationships to be central to caring and nursing and argue that emotions arise from the relationship between nurse and patient mediated by the structures of western market driven health care in which the relationship takes place.

Challenging definitions of caring

Challenging definitions of caring

More recently, Paley (2001) has disputed this whole genre of research and argued that researchers attempting to define care have taken what nurses (and others) say about caring behaviours to be what care is; that is, the research is based on claims to care rather than observed caring behaviours. Morse *et al.* (1992) also criticise these approaches, arguing that caring is too restrictive and does not encompass all that nurses do.

The value of the data in this book begins to address Paley's critiques of this literature. By using ethnography which includes participant observation and interviews, I both elicited claims to care as well as directly observed caring behaviours. And in the later chapters in this book, I also address Morse *et al.*'s (1992) point by showing that caring is more than tasks or attributes. In these empirical data, I show how caring is about relationships and being present.

Of course, nursing's claim to be a science and an art of caring is also claimed by medicine and other health care workers (Pellegrino 1983; Brewin 1993). Salvage (1990) has criticised the claim to care as a political strategy while I have argued elsewhere (Allan 2007b) that the rhetoric of a caring ideology in nursing has masked our inability as trained nurses to provide time for care. Caring as the emotional focus of nursing rather than an instrumental or practical feature of nursing practice has been criticised extensively (Dunlop 1986; Waterworth & Luker 1990; May 1990; Ashworth *et al.* 1992; Bradshaw 1995). It is argued that nurse researchers have ignored and further devalued the physical aspects of caring and delegated those activities to non-nurses while retaining the high status emotional caring for themselves. These critics suggest that while physical caring is not distinctive to nursing, caring is still a part of nursing and no less important to patients for that lack of distinctiveness. Indeed, Aldridge (1994), writing from a social work perspective, warns nurses to 'keep the technical skills in the foreground and build relationships upon them. It is more politically realistic but less destructively stressful' (1994:727). In Chapters 7 and 8 on advanced roles, the data shows that it is exactly this ability to integrate emotional and bedside or technical care that nurses working at advanced levels exploit.

Another factor framing the claim to care which has been identified recently following substantial health policy changes to the delivery of community care to patients with long-term conditions, is whether societies can afford to deliver care. Some authors have argued that many industrial countries are faced with the conundrum of reducing expenditure on care delivery while at the same time improving quality of care to meet expectations (Temmink *et al.* 2000; Allan 2007b). This pressure on resources is a very real driver for the extension of nursing roles rather than their advancement which I shall discuss in Chapter 9.

Care: a theoretical or descriptive category?

There have been attempts to define caring in order to create a universal definition applying to nursing (Watson 1988; Benner & Wrubel 1989). However, Thomas (1993) argues that care is not a theoretical category but a descriptive one which has been inconsistently defined to give the impression that it is a unified theoretical concept. She suggests using care as a descriptive category which delineates the parameters of care which carers engage in. She states: 'care as a concept reflects common-sense constructs reflecting the concrete manifestations of types of activity which society recognises as "looking after people, or people work, or people-centred work"' (Thomas 1993:665). As a descriptive category, caring is taken to have two dimensions, the material and the emotional (Graham 1993) which is given to dependent or able bodied people (Thomas 1994) by a variety of carers who may or may not establish affective relationships (Qureshi & Walker 1990). Lastly, care may be formal or informal and waged and unwaged (Thomas 1994).

A theoretical overview of caring and emotions

From this brief overview, it can be seen that caring has been strongly linked with mothering and emotion work. This means that nurses are strongly linked with mothering and emotion work through the association between nursing, caring and women's work in the home. These associations seem to be explained by the interrelationship between biological and social factors in women's lives, such as the biological need for some aspects of mothering (pregnancy, childbirth and breast feeding) and the social reproduction of western gender roles (including other aspects of mothering such as feeding, washing and teaching which are culturally seen as feminine roles but are not cross-culturally so). Caring is determined (in nursing) by these two factors along with the context of health care in which nursing takes place. But these are taken for granted assumptions about women's work. The gendered position of nursing vis-à-vis medicine (Davies 1995; Porter 1995), the nature of professions and semi-professions (Hearn 1982) and the hierarchical structures of class and ethnicity within nursing itself (Porter 1995) shape the nature of caring within nursing. Caring itself comprises those physical and psychological activities which patients, nurses and other professionals associate with caring and nursing (Bradshaw 1995; Thomas 1994). These activities are balanced according to the needs of the patient and the nurse takes her lead from the patient to care within the nurse–patient relationship (Purkiss 1996). Caring also entails emotional labour by the nurse/carer (James 1992; Smith 1992). The links between caring and emotions have formed an increasingly large section of the literature on caring and to develop the argument in the later chapters of this book, this literature on emotions needs to be discussed in the context of other perspectives on emotions and their role in health and illness.

Reflection:

Whatever field you practice in, you will care for patients. Take a short time to reflect on what you've been taught about caring during your nursing education. How central is caring to what you now do in practice? In what ways do you feel caring is innately linked to being a woman? Or do you consider caring to be a human not a gendered attribute? In other words, do men care? And lastly, can nurses claim to care above other professions?

Emotions and nursing

Emotions and nursing

One strand of the emerging nursing discourse around emotions can be traced back to Strauss *et al.* (1982) who argued that there has been a shift in health care around caring and emotions to a position where instrumental and technical care dominates the sentimental which has become invisible. In contrast in a later paper, Aldridge (1994) argues that there is a shift in nursing culture towards valuing emotional care above instrumental caring as a political stance to increase professional status.

However, Phillips (1996) points out in a review of the emotional labour in nursing literature, that while it is argued by nurses that they provide emotional care and assert that this is what patients want, what many researchers have found is that nurses are mostly engaged in instrumental care and the delivery of routine tasks. The meaning of emotional labour, the context in which nurses claim to care and do emotional labour, and the value given to this work are therefore contentious issues which influence nursing's claims to professional status and its unique place in health care.

Emotional labour

Within nursing, Smith (1992) used a definition of emotion which is derived from Hochschild's (1983) work on emotional labour. Smith (1992) focused specifically on emotional labour in nursing as a way of naming the elusive nature of care. Emotional labour is the 'management of feeling to create a publicly observable facial and bodily display; emotional labour is sold for a wage' (Hochschild 1983:7). Selling emotional labour for a wage devalues emotions which become unrecognised within the workplace. Emotion work and management are used interchangeably by Hochschild to mean the same acts as emotional labour but done in the private context which have exchange value. Hochschild's definition of emotion is discussed later in the chapter to show the influence of the main theories of emotions on her theory of emotional labour. Smith's findings suggest that the emotional labour expected of nurses by managers is hidden and devalued in the health care context.

Emotional closeness or distance?

Another strand in the historical development of the nursing discourse around emotions can be seen in research into the nurse–patient relationship. Researchers have emphasised feelings such as closeness (Peplau 1969; Meutzal 1988); empathy and trust (Gardner & Wheeler 1981; Watson 1988); positive unconditional regard (Strang 1982) and support (Gardner & Wheeler 1987) within the nurse–patient relationship. This tradition has been influenced by Rogers' ideas on unconditional positive regard forming the basis of the therapeutic relationship (1951; 1975). The nature of the nurse–patient relationship has also been discussed in terms of feelings developing between the patient and nurse through the use of self (Uys 1980; Meutzal 1988; Barber 1991).

In contrast, nursing as therapy was criticised by Savage in the 1990s in a study into the nature of new forms of nursing in the 1990s, the 'new nursing' which was a resurgence of the value of professional nursing. Savage (1995) found that while physical and emotional closeness and intimacy are values promoted by the 'new nursing', nurses do not necessarily facilitate relationships of 'emotional intensity' with their patients. Emotional distance is a characteristic of nurse–patient relationships which can be described as close but nevertheless have a varying degree of detachment. Savage (1995:123) interpreted Peplau's (1969) writings to propose a closeness which includes an emotional distance. This emotional distance is achieved through nurses working to construct a caring environment which is therapeutic for patients 'without great personal cost for the nurse' (Savage 1995:124).

Morse (1991) has delineated the strategies with which nurses and patients develop and inhibit the emotional links in the nurse–patient relationship. Other researchers have focused on patients' positive feelings towards nurses, such as kindness (Champion *et al.* 1987) and virtue while also pointing out that these positive feelings felt by patients towards nurses were also associated with patients' views of nurses as lacking knowledge, being powerless and dependent.

Why are emotions nursing's business?

Unfortunately, within the literature on the nature of emotions in the nurse–patient relationship there is no discussion of the historical context of emotions. This means that emotions are presented as the natural concern of nurses to justify their occupational status as expressive specialists (May 1990). This literature firstly gives the impression that emotions have emerged as the 'natural' business of nursing and nurses because of the historical association between women, caring and love. Secondly, the Rogerian influence on this school (which emphasises unconditional positive regard and love) has meant that positive emotions in the nurse–patient relationship have been emphasised. In contrast, the psychoanalytic school believes that love exists with hate. For example, Buber (cited by Kirschenbaum & Henderson 1989) disagrees with Rogers on unconditional positive regard/reciprocity. He argues that the therapist–client relationship is inherently unequal because the reason for the relationship in the first place is the client's distress. Therefore, such a relationship can never be equal or reciprocal and therefore the therapist can never hold the patient in unconditional positive regard. The same criticisms can be made of claims by Meutzal (1988) to a reciprocal relationship between nurses and patients. Fabricius (1991a) argues that both positive and negative feelings need to be acknowledged and utilised to be therapeutic. In nursing, consequently there are differences in interpretation between Rogerian perspectives in nursing theory (Barber 1991; Ersser 1997) and psychoanalytic perspective (Fabricius 1991a; 1991b) around how effectively the nurse can act therapeutically in her use of self. I will now turn to a brief overview of the two main theories on emotions which have influenced nursing theories.

Reflection:

Reflect on how far you agree with the idea that emotions are integral to nursing practice. Indeed, is it possible to deliver emotional care within a busy NHS setting?

Theories of emotions

Theories of emotions

There have been two main theories of emotions which have been influential in health care, the organismic (Mitchell 1974) and the interactionist (Hochschild 1983).

Organismic theory of emotions

The organismic view of emotions emerged from the work of 19th century writers such as Darwin (1955), Freud (1964) and James (1922). While emotions were understood by Darwin as biological drives, and by James as the brain's conscious reaction to instinctual visceral changes, Freud's understanding of emotions shows an awareness of the interplay between biology and the social environment through unconscious and conscious processes, a move away from biological determinism with which he is associated (Mitchell 1974; Hochschild 1983). I use unconscious here to describe processes of inner thoughts and feelings which are not brought to consciousness (awareness) (Badcock 1992).

Our unconscious normally represses emotions but they emerge through conscious thought, introspection or through unconscious slips of the tongue (Mitchell 1974), or expressed emotions such as anger; or are somatised through illness (Erskine & Judd 1994). The relationship between the unconscious and the conscious in the realm of emotions is that of the experience and the expression of emotions.

We may experience an emotion unconsciously or experience and express it consciously (Craib 1995). The extent to which one influences the other is debated in sociology between those who argue that the unconscious experience can exist without the expression or be revealed unwittingly or through introspection (Craib 1995) and those who believe that the expression determines the experience of the emotion (Jackson 1993; Duncombe & Marsden 1993). In other words, do I feel an emotion if I cannot name it or am unaware of it?

One further aspect of Freud's theory of the unconscious is pertinent to further development of ideas in this book. Freud believed that society was the result of our ability to repress emotions which were antisocial, through the unconscious (Sayers 1991; Badcock 1992). If expressed, such emotions would disrupt society. Displays of emotions therefore represent conscious thoughts which are socially acceptable and individually tolerable, while antisocial emotions are either repressed by the unconscious or consciously suppressed by the individual.[2] These conscious and unconscious processes are how society emerges from the individual: uncomfortable or unacceptable emotions are

---

[2] Badcock (1992) discussion of the pleasure and reality principles are useful on this point. While the unconscious may repress uncomfortable feelings by the pleasure principle, it is also driven by the reality principle and therefore repression can cease and uncomfortable feelings rise to the conscious.

repressed through unconscious and conscious thoughts to enable individuals to interact in groups. Both unconscious and conscious thoughts and feelings have meaning within the individual's subjectivity or personal history as they are shaped by early family experiences (Mitchell 1974; Chodorow 1989; Craib 1995).

The importance of Freud's theory of emotions for this book lies in his theory of the unconscious and conscious emotional life, and the strength which emotions and their repression or suppression arouse for staff and patients.

Freud's ideas have been criticised and his theory of an unconscious mental life denied by many within sociology. However, there appears to be a greater willingness to discuss his ideas and apply them to social theory (Connell 1987; Figlio 1987; Hunt 1989; Badcock 1992; Craib 1995; Lupton 1995) as Orbach (1999:12) suggests, because his theory can 'enhance our approach to social problems'. While Hochschild (1983) does not utilise Freud's understanding of the unconscious, she uses Freud's idea of the 'signal function' of emotions to define emotions as a biologically given sense orientation to action; that is, emotional senses orientate through their signal function to act when stimulated. An emotional sense of anger alerts the individual to a feeling emerging from interactions in the environment and the individual expresses anger in action. However, Hochschild (1983) argues that feelings are also socially shaped through cultural rules (feeling rules) about emotional display and through cognitive processes in perception. She develops these ideas from Goffman (1959) and symbolic interactionism.

(Symbolic) Interactionist theory of emotions

The interactionist view of emotions derives from Dewey (1922), Gerth & Wright-Mills (1964) and Goffman (1959). The interactionist view of emotions is that emotions can only be understood in their social context; the social context shapes feelings (Dewey 1922). Gerth & Wright Mills (1964) argued that emotions comprise gesture, conscious experience and a physiological process. Goffman (1959) developed Gerth & Wright Mills' theory of emotions through studying the ways in which social beings understand feeling rules through displays of feeling and gesture. He argued that 'true or real attitudes, beliefs & emotions can be ascertained only indirectly' (1959:14) through the meaning the actor attaches to a behaviour or the involuntary expressed behaviour. Therefore, every act can be interpreted by the observer and the actor as having a motive which the actor tries to convey through the act.

His use of language, such as act, actor, dramaturgical, and his failure to clarify where the motive originates from, leads the more psychoanalytically disposed reader to interpret Goffman's work as dealing with the surface act rather than the inner meaning. Hochschild (1983:216) argues that '... for Goffman, acting is surface acting. The actor's mental focus is on the slope of a shoulder, the angle of a glance, or the tightness of a smile, not on any inner feeling to which such gestures might correspond. Deep acting is not empirically alive in Goffman's work'. And recognising this lack in Goffman's work, Hochschild (1983) includes deep acting as part of emotional labour by drawing on Freud's theory of emotions as signal functions. Deep acting works by either exhorting a feeling or by making indirect use of a trained imagination for a wage or reward as in nursing (Hochschild 1983). Hochschild (1983) emphasised that Goffman argued that humans acted behaviourally, motivated by social rules and groups, as opposed to Freud who argued that feelings determined behaviour.

Applying organicist and interactionist theories of emotions

Both Freud's and Goffman's work have been widely interpreted by different researchers. Hunt (1989) argues (from a psychoanalytic perspective) that there are varying degrees of value placed on the relationship between feelings and the unconscious in shaping human behaviour. Hunt (1989:19) argues that the symbolic interactionist has 'no unconscious mental life. Although his or her world is meaningful, its significance is derived from the surface, interactional level of experience'.

On the other hand, Branaman (1997) argues that Goffman's definitions of self are contradictory. The self is both a social product yet has an unsocialised component; that is, it acts socially from social pressure and simultaneously from inner drives which arise in feelings. The self acts both in roles which are determined by cultural rules and *yet also* determined by the self.

Although both Freud and Goffman believed that the social context was important, it was Freud who developed a theory of psychological subjectivity (meaning) which explored the influence of an individual's feelings on behaviour. Essentially, the organismic and interactionist views of emotions have been presented in the literature as contradictory. The organismic is presented as biological. The interactionist is presented as largely social, that is, an emotion becomes an emotion when it is socially constructed to be so and interpreted by the individual and the group as such through cognition and language (Duncombe & Marsden 1993; Craib 1995).

The interactionist school has been the most influential within nursing theory on caring and emotions (James 1992; Smith 1992; Froggart 1998; Spiers 1998). The organismic school has been more influential within medicine (Balint 1964; Main 1968; Elder & Samuel 1987) and associated professions such as counselling within health care (Ross 1995; Hunt & Monach 1997; Pietroni 1993; Erskine & Judd 1994). A recent development of the organismic perspective is the emotions in organisations approach which facilitates organisations and groups within them to deal with stress engendered by caring by focusing on the 'unconscious' at work (Obholzer 1993; Obholzer & Zagier Roberts 1994; Obholzer 2003). There are only two nurses writing from an organismic perspective currently: Barber (1991), a Gestalt therapist influenced by Rogers (1967) and Fabricius (1991a; 1991b), a psychoanalyst.

Psychoanalytic approaches in nursing

Psycho-analytic approaches

Psychoanalytic theories of emotions are based on Freud's theory of the unconscious.[3] Two principal ideas from this theory are useful in exploring the effects of emotions on clinical interactions in the context of reproductive technologies:

Freud's theory of the unconscious:

1. the unconscious repression of painful emotions
2. the psychosexual development of children and the importance of generative capability for adults.

---

[3] In the following discussion I draw on more recent theoretical developments of Freud's ideas as Freud's original ideas have been substantially critiqued and reworked.

A theoretical overview of caring and emotions

The unconscious repression of emotions

The unconscious is the site where anti-social emotions are repressed, that is, not made conscious or raised to awareness (Mitchell 1974; Barber 1991). These emotions are most commonly aggressive or sexual and can exert an influence on behaviour especially in times of anxiety or stress while remaining unconscious (Barber 1991; Fabricius 1991b; Ross 1995). Fabricius (1991b) has described the psychoanalytic perspective as concerned with 'processes which involve opposing forces and conflicts' (1991a:135); these opposing forces are emotions in Fabricius' view. Emotional conflicts arise from the interplay between biology, social conditioning and internal psychic processes unconsciously and consciously (Mitchell 1974; Tong 1994; Fabricius 1991b).[4] For example, consciously, a nurse knows she must be polite to a demanding patient but unconsciously, she may feel anger towards the patient which she represses. Her repressed anger may be obvious in her body language but she is not aware that she is angry. These internal, unconscious conflicts are present in human interactions and, of course, between staff and patients, becoming evident in slips of the tongue, jokes and sarcasm (Ross 1995). Ross (1995) has suggested that in areas such as gynaecology, where staff deal with primitive, unconscious emotions surrounding death, life and sexuality, anxiety is aroused constantly. Primitive in this instance means the feelings which are evoked in the id deep within the unconscious.[5] A nurse may, on the other hand, consciously be angry with a patient but suppress her anger. This conscious suppression is a different process to repression. The nurse is consciously aware of her feelings although she does not express them (Badcock 1992).

4 I have used the term emotion within a psychoanalytic perspective rather than a biological or cognitive, following Mitchell (1974), Chodorow (1989), Fabricius (1991a) and Menzies (1970).

5 According to Freud's drive theory, id is the focus of the instinctual drives which shape internal emotions. These drives are often described as primitive as the id is anti-social. Ego is the rational internal control over the id as the drives, being anti-social and concerned with aggression and sex, are destructive. Internal psychic conflict arises between ego and id which Superego resolves to a degree. Superego is the conscience which is largely imposed from the external world (Chodorow 1989). In Chodorow's view, in Object-relations theory, it is the superego which provides the influence of the social in the development of a child's psychic world. There is, in other words, less emphasis on drives and more emphasis on interactions with the outside world particularly the primary carers (Chodorow 1989). Gender, in Chodorow's analysis, is shaped through the influence of superego which includes the expecta-tions, norms and values associated with gender development. In a patriarchal society, the female superego is weaker, more dependent than the male and this is seen as psychically normal.

Managing intimacy and emotions

Traditionally in both medicine and nursing, feelings have been both ignored and denied and clinical practitioners encouraged to distance themselves from feelings in case they contaminate the clinical interaction and prevent efficient medical and nursing practice (Clifford 1998; Murray Parkes 1998). However, infertility arouses painful, primitive emotions because it touches on our experiences of sexuality and birth. It becomes necessary for fertility nurses to both repress and suppress emotions if they are to function in socially appropriate ways at work.

Menzies (1970) and Fabricius (1991a; 1991b) argue that a denial of feelings has led to defences against the anxieties aroused by the awareness of emotions in nursing practice. In other words, even though nurses have been encouraged to ignore and deny feelings, this has not meant that feelings have ceased to exist. Instead, anxiety has been channelled into ways of working which inhibit close contact and connection with patients in an attempt to deny feelings. Menzies called these ways of working social defence systems.[6] Recently, the focus on nurse–patient interactions advocated by patient allocation and primary nursing has led to an awareness of feelings, the approach advocated by the nursing as therapy school (Meutzal 1988; Ersser 1997). But Fabricius (1991a) argues that there has been a lack of any significant accompanying change in nurse–patient relationships. Nurses have not been able to connect emotionally with patients generally and have remained distant in a defence against the anxiety aroused by confronting painful emotions. The social defence systems have remained despite the ideological and theoretical advocacy of therapeutic nursing (Fabricius 1991a). Barber's (1991) description of his hospitalisation as a patient in which he described the continued existence of defences against

---

6 Menzies' social defence systems in the case of nursing involve :
- splitting of the nurse–patient relationship through reduced contact
- depersonalisation and denial of significance of the individual patient for the nurse
- detachment or denial of feelings towards patient
- elimination of decisions through a ritual task performance
- checks and counterchecks to reduce responsibility for decision making
- collusive social redistribution of responsibility and irresponsibility
- purposeful obscurity in the formal distribution of responsibility
- reduced impact of responsibility by delegation to superiors
- idealisation and underestimation of personal development possibilities
- avoidance of change

Menzies (1970)

anxiety is a powerful reminder of the strength of social defence systems caused by emotions in the nurse–patient relationship. However, Savage (1995) has argued that there has been patchy change in the types of nurse–patient relationships particularly in Nursing Development Units (NDUs).

The denial of emotions in clinical practice is an issue recognised by practitioners utilising the Balint method of GP consultations (Balint 1957; Elder & Samuel 1987) and psychosexual nursing (Clifford *et al.* 2000). Balint[7] used a psychoanalytic approach to clinical interactions between doctors and patients. The key insights gained from this approach are that emotions do exist, that they are often repressed conjointly by patient and doctor, that they can be acknowledged through honest and natural communication and worked with to produce change in patient behaviour (Elder & Samuel 1987).

Applying these insights to nursing,[8] Clifford (1998:155) has said: 'Involvement supported by professional self-reflection, however, can give us the means to stay with the pain evoked in us by our patients, rather than defend ourselves against it'. Similarly, Fabricius (1991a:137) aims to 'help them (nurses) to become more aware, both of their feelings, fears and impulses and of the defences they use in order not to be aware' in nursing practice. The rationale for acknowledging the unconscious repression of painful and antisocial emotions is that the social defence systems which are erected to avoid awareness, divert energies from caring, to 'meeting unconscious needs for survival and the reduction of anxiety' (Ross 1995:210). The primary task of nursing therefore becomes maintaining the social defence systems rather than caring which nursing theorists consider to be the role of nursing. The primary task was maintaining the social defence system through the management of emotions rather than caring for patients and their needs as suggested in the activity of 'nursing the clinic and the doctor' which is discussed in Chapter 4.

---

[7] Eric Balint was a psychoanalyst who worked with general practitioners at the Tavistock Clinic in the 1950s.

[8] There have been three main developments of psychodynamic nursing in the UK. The Balint school has been utilised by psychosexual nurses involved with psychosexual counselling, see Selby (1990), the Cassell Hospital which under Thomas Main after the Second World War started psychodynamic nursing as part of a therapeutic community for mentally ill patients, see Barnes E, Griffiths P, Ord J & Wells D (1998) and Menzies important paper in 1957 (Menzies 1970) from which Fabricius, a nurse and psychoanalyst developed her ideas on applying psychoanalysis to nursing (1991a; 1991b; 1995).

Managing intimacy and emotions

Non-caring

Non-caring

The idea that nurses are non-caring is uncomfortable for nurses. So much so that Leininger (1990) argues that non-caring practices will be legally challenged and virtually eradicated in the future. This is rather naïve given the evidence of non-caring in the British literature. The nursing discourse on caring has assumed from its humanist base that all nursing care actions are well-intentioned (Noddings 1984; Watson 1988) and have a more or less positive effect (Ersser 1997). However, the data from this study shows that nurses engage in activities which are non-caring. There is a small amount of literature emerging on non-caring which begins to challenge the hegemony of caring as an ideology within nursing. There are several explanations for non-caring actions which will be briefly considered here and analysed with the data in later chapters.

Explanations for non-caring

The first explanation for non-caring is that the caring discourse has ignored the realities of nursing work (Clifford 1995) and the emotional stresses of dealing with dependent patients under varying degrees of stress (Menzies 1970).

There is plenty of evidence that nurses do not care (Waterworth & Luker 1990; May 1990; Ashworth *et al.* 1992; Armstrong-Esther *et al.* 1994) and that the structures in which care takes place in the National Health Service (NHS) militate against caring. Examples include patients submitting out of fear of getting into trouble (Waterworth & Luker 1990) or the extent of routinised, superficial and task orientated nursing care which focuses on inconsequential talk (May 1990). The reality of care work is that it involves physical labour and hard work, long hours, emotional turmoil and moral debate (Daniels 1987). In this case, the demands of caring might be a justified excuse for non-caring.

Secondly, the interpretation of non-caring depends on the definition of caring. Davies (1995) suggests that caring may be 'knowing' someone is there to respond if asked. In this case, nurses might not appear caring because they have not acted; but viewing caring as a response to demand, they might be seen as passively waiting for a patient to ask for care and, therefore, caring. Thirdly, Gorovitz (1994) argues that patients expect caring in the medical context to include both a good outcome and a good experience.

However, they prefer a good outcome. Therefore, instrumental and efficient caring is more important than the emotional side of caring.

Lastly, Purkiss (1996) argues that judging nursing care is not a question of 'good or bad caring' but of asking why did this happen? She argues non-caring arises from the social identities which patients and nurses construct from past experience and current interactions. 'Good' nursing is not good *per se* but is expected from the identities ascribed to nurses which patients hold. Patients will maintain their identities of nurses by making excuses in the face of apparent non-caring. Patients also use their own behaviour to construct nurses' identities by having patient identities which they act out. Likewise, nurses construct their own identities. Non-caring in this sense is socially constructed through the nurse–patient relationship.

The contributions that these theories of emotions can make to caring within nursing are explored in later chapters of this book. I conclude this chapter by suggesting a conceptual framework for analysing emotions and caring which is then illustrated in Chapter 4.

A possible theory of emotions for nursing practice

A theory of emotions

Data from study 1 suggested an organicist rather than an interactionist perspective. Patients' descriptions of infertility as a life-crisis with profound emotional effects, and the ways in which staff managed emotion in the clinics suggested a psychological or internal level, an organicist perspective, shaped by the demands of the external environment which could include the demands of the system or the hospital organisation. As Craib (1995:155) says: 'Individuals, people – men and women – are by definition engaged in at least two interlocking forms of emotional work: the internal work of coping with contradiction, conflict and ambivalence and the external work of reconciling what goes on inside with what one is supposed or allowed to feel'. I argue that staff managed feelings in their attempts to reconcile internal feelings with the realities of their external working environment. Acting was a feature of behaviours within the clinic but was not sufficient to explain the contradictions in the data. I agree with Craib (1995) that emotions are dynamic and more than just social constructions dependent on the context in which they are expressed for meaning.

Therefore, I use the term emotional work as Craib (1995) uses it, to refer to emotional effort, rather than distinguish between private and paid forms of emotional work or emotional labour. I use the term emotional management or managing emotions to describe the defences that staff used to achieve this control. I argue that staff controlled emotions generated by infertility as a defence against anxiety rather than as a response to the demands of capital as Hochschild (1983) and Smith (1992) argue. In addition to their emotional defences, I have suggested that in 'nursing the clinic and doctor' nurses responded to the demands of powerful managerial and professional forces. Staff's defences against anxiety, their internal work, mutually constituted the social systems in the unit which were in turn shaped by the hospital environment, the biomedical culture and traditional working relationships between medicine and nursing, their external work.

Theories of emotions are attempts to understand where mind, body and society meet. Sociological theories have not analysed feelings in the context of whether they are comfortable or uncomfortable internally or as an unconscious experience. The emotional labour theory, developed from symbolic interaction-ism, has focused on caring as labour and the constraints on private emotions which caring entails when performed by a wage in public. While Smith (1992) recognises that negative emotions can be utilised as part of emotional labour, e.g. 'old school' ward sisters evoking fear in student nurses, the literature on the therapeutic nature of the nurse–patient relationship has concentrated on the positive feelings within the relationship and ignored the negative feelings arising out of interactions with patients. Feelings have been idealised because nurses' anger towards their patients arouses uncomfortable feelings (Fabricius 1991a).

Summarising this chapter:

Now write a short summary of what has been presented in this chapter on caring and the theories of emotions using the following bullet points:

- Why is caring seen as central to nursing and midwifery?
- Do you think it's central?
- What are emotions and why are they important?
- How do you deal with your emotions at work?

You might like to discuss your ideas with a colleague.

Chapter 3
The experience of infertility

In Chapter 2, I introduced the main theories on caring in nursing and ended with a discussion of two theories of emotions. I suggested that understanding the ways that emotions influence caring is a useful way to think about how caring is experienced for both nurse and patient in the nurse–patient relationship. In addition to the role of emotions in ordinary nurse–patient relationships, emotions are integral to the experience of infertility for patients. Two different traditions have provided explanations of why and how emotions are so powerful for infertile people. These traditions are psychology and psychoanalysis. Therefore, in this chapter I provide an overview of the experience of infertility from psychological and psychoanalytic perspectives.

Reflection:

While you read this chapter, think of a patient or couple with whom you have worked and consider whether the research outlined here has any relevance for their experience.

Early writing on infertility: Barbara Menning

Early writing on infertility

Some of the most influential, early work on infertility (perhaps the most influential) which describes the experience of infertility was by Menning (1977; 1980) and it is sufficiently important to refer to in some depth.[9] She describes infertility as a life crisis, a period of disequilibrium. This is characterised by a threat to life goals

[9] Her ideas are based on her experience as an infertility counsellor and her experience of working with Resolve, the American organisation which offers support groups and counselling.

which is insoluble in the immediate future; it over taxes the resources of the person(s) affected and it may reawaken unsolved psychological problems from the past (Menning 1980). On top of these experiences, the crisis of infertility recurs again and again in cycles of hope, loss and despair. Menning argues that this recurrence can result in adaptive or maladaptive behaviours which elicit coping strategies (Menning 1980). Menning argues that infertile couples experience a syndrome of feelings as they attempt to resolve the infertility crisis. She describes these feelings quite specifically in order:

- surprise
- denial
- anger
- isolation
- guilt
- grief
- resolution.

This order is important as Menning's theory is a staged theory of grieving where one stage succeeds the other; missing stages can be harmful to eventual resolution. Menning (1977) compares her stages of infertility crisis to Kubler-Ross' stages of dying (1973).

She suggests that the loss an infertile couple experiences, while it cannot be felt concretely, is the loss of the imagined child. This potential loss is not always recognised; it may be socially unspeakable, it can be uncertain, it may not be socially valued as a loss and the infertile couple may have no social support system. This imagined loss is as great as the concrete loss at death.

While the data in study 1 from patients' interviews showed that infertility produces periods of uncertainty and is extremely painful, Menning bases her observations and her syndrome of feelings on a model of grieving which assumes resolution. Menning (1977:116) describes the stage of resolution as characterised by the naming of the feeling which is causing distress, talking about the feeling as honestly as possible and finding relief from the feeling before moving on to a new feeling state. A block to resolution may occur in any of the stages of the crisis but when resolution is finally accomplished, the infertility is experienced as a 'sweet sadness' rather than bitterness. This successful end to the crisis is achieved through the acceptance of an alternative lifestyle (Menning 1980).

In contrast, Raphael-Leff (1991) and Pines (1993), two psycho-analysts, suggest that the resolution of loss is not a final endpoint, something to be achieved or experienced. Instead, resolution may include ambivalence surrounding the diminishing of the intensity of the feelings of loss, i.e. it may be difficult to 'end' the infertility experience as that implies saying goodbye to the possibility of becoming a biological parent even if this means continuing to experience painful feelings. The resolution of loss includes the acceptance of an alternative lifestyle. They argue that, rather than discussing this ambivalence in terms of loss, at this point infertile couples can be encouraged to think about roles which society has not encouraged and which may now be possible.

Reflection:

How did the patient or couple you worked with resolve their infertility? Do you think resolution is possible?

Psychological explorations of the experience of infertility

Psychological explorations

Apart from Menning, there is an extensive psychological literature on the experience of infertility. This literature has traditionally viewed infertility as an abnormal state which is stressful and requires psychological adjustment (Frank 1989; Davis & Dearman 1991; Prattke & Gass-Sternas 1993). At the same time it has suggested that the answer to unexplained infertility lies in the woman's psychopathology (Sandelowski 1990; Greil 1997; Christie 1998). The psychoanalytic school contributed to this tendency in psychological research until recently (Christie 1998). Consequently, much of the older psychological research focused on the abnormalities within the infertile couple and searched for psychological and psychosomatic causes of infertility. The assumption that infertility both causes or is caused by an abnormal psychological state means that the negative attributes of infertility are well documented in the psychological literature and include: isolation (Christianson 1986); lack of control (McCormick 1980; Milne 1988); emotional disequilibrium (McCormick 1980); altered self-image (for the worse); guilt;

resentment; and marital stresses and disharmony (Hirsch and Hirsch 1989; Millard 1991; Halman *et al.* 1994).

The stressful nature of infertility and ARTs

More recently, researchers have acknowledged the innately stressful nature of both infertility and infertility treatments and investigations and have explored the similarities between infertile and fertile experiences of reproduction (Sandelowski 1990; Greil 1997; Christie 1998). In other words, researchers have been slow to accept that to grieve and show distress is a normal reaction to infertility and does not mean that there is necessarily a connection between the infertility and the woman's psychological state.

Some studies have attempted to predict criteria for candidate selection to IVF, egg donation and AID programmes (Greenfield & Haseltine 1986; Prattke & Gass-Sternas 1993; Eugster & Vingerhoets 1999) based on infertile couples' experiences and perceived coping responses to stressful treatments. For example, Carr *et al.* (1990) developed predictive measurements of the psychological difficulty men wanting to undergo AID might have if offered treatment. This research has also included the success-fully treated infertile parent now that there are many more children born from ARTs. These studies investigate the ability of the infertile parent to be a good enough parent (MRC Working Party on Children Conceived by IVF 1990; Jones 1994; Golombok *et al.* 1995). Psychological predictors are used to measure parenting skills and point to society's concern about the ethics of ARTs. Eugster & Vingerhoets (1999) undertook a major review of the research into psychological reactions of women before entering IVF, during IVF treatments, and after both successful and unsuccessful IVF treatment. They argued that, in general, couples who enter IVF programmes are well adjusted, but find the experience of IVF stressful. IVF parents experience more stress during pregnancy compared with non-IVF parents, and IVF mothers self-report a higher quality of parent–child relationship than mothers with naturally conceived children.

Quality of life

In other papers comparing women's experiences of successful and unsuccessful infertility treatment (both IVF and GIFT), Weaver *et al.* (1993), Leiblum *et al.* (1998), Malin *et al.* (2001), Hjelmstedt

(2003), McMahon *et al.* (2003) and Hjelmstedt *et al.* (2004) make significant contributions to understanding the complex ways in which infertility treatments affect pregnancy, birth and parenthood. Weaver *et al.* (1993) sampled 20 couples who conceived through IVF/GIFT and used questionnaires to measure quality of life, parents' feelings about their babies, and child-rearing attitudes. IVF parents showed no differences from non-IVF parents in respect to marital adjustment and emotional health, but did give higher ratings for their feelings about their babies, and were generally more 'overprotective'. This finding is important, as it suggests that the notion of 'overprotective' behaviour needs to be explored further. Leiblum *et al.* (1998), using a 'life after IVF' questionnaire to compare childless women (n = 18), IVF mothers (n = 41) and non-IVF mothers (n = 16), found that childless women were significantly less satisfied with their lives than IVF mothers or mothers who conceived naturally. Using a survey questionnaire on 3000 women in Finland (response rate = 74%), Malin *et al.* (2001) found that women responded well to open-ended and semi-structured questions about their satisfaction with infertility examinations and treatment. The birth of a baby was the most common reason for satisfaction, and the most common reason for dissatisfaction was unsatisfactory encounters with medical staff. Again, this finding needs to be explored to understand how medical encounters were substandard and what could be done to improve them. There is a dearth of literature concerning women's views of encounters with midwives in the maternity services when IVF has been successful.

McMahon *et al.* (2003) matched groups of IVF parents who had successfully conceived with those who conceived naturally, for psychosocial adjustment. Their work contributes to a growing body of research that demonstrates normal psychosocial adjustment in parents conceiving through IVF, rather than more positive adjustment that earlier studies claimed to show (Golombok *et al.*, 1996). In Hjelmstedt's (2003) first study, a comparison of 57 IVF mothers and 55 IVF fathers with 43 non-IVF mothers and 39 non-IVF fathers, a measurement scale was used to focus on anxiety during early and late pregnancy. They discovered that IVF mothers had more positive experiences of pregnancy than non-IVF mothers, and that IVF fathers were worried about birth injuries. In a second study, Hjelmstedt *et al.* (2004) compared IVF parents (mothers = 55; fathers = 53) with non-IVF parents (mothers = 40; fathers = 36), using a self-rating scale to measure parenting stress and marital relationship during pregnancy, and at two and six months after birth. It was found that the inability to conceive continued to affect the current lives of IVF parents. Negative feelings related to infertility were not easily overcome among IVF parents. This has implications for provision of a 'space' for women to relate this sensitive information early in the pregnancy so that care can be tailored accordingly.

The psychopathology of infertility

Over the 1990s a subtle shift in perspective took place within the psychological literature which means that explanations of the psychopathology of the infertile person and the negative psychological consequences of infertility are not always so prominent in psychological research. An example is Boivin's work (2008) which suggests that infertile couples who stop treatment are less likely to divorce than the general population and can successfully find new purposes in life to survive the trauma of infertility treatment failure. Christie's 1998 paper and Greil's 1997 literature review were important in assisting this shift (Koropatrick 1993; Schmidt *et al.* 2005; Cousineau *et al.* 2006; Rossen & Gruber 2007). However, the language some authors use continues to reflect their underlying assumptions that psychopathology remains a possible cause of infertility. So, for example, Bringhenti *et al.* (1997) have shown that infertile women have higher rates of satisfaction with their marital relationships but conclude 'Infertile women *do not necessarily* show signs of psychological maladjustment. Their level of state-anxiety can be considered a situational response to treatment stress' (1997:431) (my italics).

However what is largely unacknowledged about the stressful nature of infertility for women in this literature is the importance of motherhood for some women and not for others. There is little debate over the question of whether the desire for a child is socially or biologically shaped. Indeed, the Charity More to Life (http://www.infertilitynetworkuk.com/moretolife/) argue that the involuntary childless state is seen and judged as psychologically abnormal due to a thwarted biological or social drive and therefore requires investigation. They provide support for those who choose not to investigate reasons for childlessness as well as those who voluntarily choose not to have children.

As a patient, I was conscious that I felt I was collapsing from the weight of my emotions and that I was keen to maintain 'face' in front of the professionals so as to appear calm and normal. Yet I felt at the same time that my response was normal – my husband and I were undergoing a life-changing experience and stress and distress were perfectly normal. However I don't remember anyone saying that to me until I went into psychotherapy. It was in psychotherapy that I encountered some empathy with my situation and an explanation of why infertility seemed so emotionally traumatic. As can be seen in Chapter 6, the women I interviewed also experienced powerful emotions which seemed life threatening.

Therefore, while the psychological literature can inform fertility nurses in understanding the experience of infertile people undergoing ARTs and can assist nurses to assess patients' levels of stress and distress and intervene when appropriate and refer to counselling, it does not help fertility nurses understand the reason for these powerful emotions. I have found Chodorow's (1989) work particularly useful in understanding the role and influence of emotions in fertility nursing practice because she offers a way of understanding how infertility may be socially and psychologically shaped through her re-working of Freud's theory of sexuality. Chodorow (1989) argues that psychoanalytic feminism offers a way to think about both the social organisation and the psychology of sex and gender, and the ways in which individuals and groups engage in emotional work. Chodorow suggests that : 'Freud gives us a theory concerning how people – women and men – become gendered and sexed, how femininity and masculinity develop' (1989:176). It is the development of gender and sex that holds the key to understanding how deeply infertility affects both men and women.

Reflection:

What indicators of stress have you noticed in the patient or couple you are considering?

Psychosexual development and generative capability

Psychosexual development

Within the psychoanalytic perspective, the psychosexual development of children has been discussed in relation to mothering and caring (Chodorow 1989) as a process whereby girls learn to be feminine and dependent on others, and boys to be masculine and to separate from others. There have, of course, been disagreements as to the extent of the biological, psychological and social influences on mothering as Chodorow herself points out. A worry is that by aligning women with caring, we may reproduce inequality, given that caring is devalued as a paid occupation and seen as natural and therefore unskilled, domestic work (see Chapter 2). Infantile sexual development, and in particular the Oedipus complex, the castration complex and penis envy and the unconscious (explained in Chapter 2), the key concepts of psychoanalysis, are contentious as they can imply identification with same-sex parents, rejection of homosexuality and reinforcement of patriarchal gendered roles.

The classical Oedipal complex is based on Oedipus' murder of his father and appropriation of his father's place as his mother's husband (I have taken this interpretation from Badcock 1992). Freud argued that boys unconsciously desired their mothers and competed unsuccessfully against their fathers. Through the fear of castration, the castration complex which boys witnessed in girls' lack of a penis, boys rejected their desire for their mothers, identified with their fathers and repressed sexual desire until adolescence when they became attached sexually to a woman who replaced their primary sexual attachment. Girls experience penis envy as they realise that they have been castrated and reject their mothers, for being castrated like them, and want to have a child by their fathers. The centrality of the Oedipal and the castration complexes and penis envy remained at the root of sexual development for boys and girls for Freud.

However, the Oedipus and the castration complexes and penis envy as Freud intended them are patriarchal constructs (Sayers 1991). Critics have argued that boys and girls do indeed have sexual feelings towards their parents but that the primary attachment is the maternal one which for both sexes has to be abandoned (Chodorow 1989; Sayers 1991). However, for boys the primary sexual object remains heterosexual while for girls, it is originally homosexual and becomes, largely, heterosexual. While girls remain attached to other women more easily throughout their lives, they form sexual attachments with men to have children. As Chodorow (1989:69) argues 'Because her first love object is a woman, a girl, in order to attain her proper heterosexual orientation, must transfer her primary object choice to her father and men'.

Challenging Freud's theories

Mitchell (1974), Chodorow (1989), Tong (1994) and Sayers (1991) agree that Freud's early theories on sexual development during childhood have produced anger among feminists for their misogynistic and sexist interpretations of sexual development.

Of course Freud was writing in the late 19th and early 20th centuries at a time of male dominance or patriarchy. Chodorow (1989) defines patriarchy as 'male domination' and Weedon (1997) argues that in patriarchal societies power benefits men over women and that this exists 'in the institutions and social practices of our society and cannot be explained by the intentions, good or bad, of individual men or women' (1997:3). Historically, men dominated women through social structures which restricted women's access to and control over material resources (Evans 1996). The gender imbalance in the nursing workforce is a good example of how women were historically restricted to certain spheres of social and economic activity; namely in the case of nursing, one which had little control over health care resources and spending (Carpenter 1993). Evans suggests that this definition of patriarchy is no longer valid as there are many experiences of patriarchy which relate to the differences between women as much as the differences between men and women. Again, nursing and medicine's relationship is a good example of Evans' point here which is complex. Individual doctors may not intentionally oppress individual nurses (although some may!); but equally, women doctors may be more oppressive towards female nurses than male doctors.

In relation to the social and psychological gender development of boys and girls, patriarchal societies restrict who mothers in terms of gender. For example, in the fertility field, this is clearly seen in the debates over who is 'fit to mother' in the proposed

Human Fertilisation and Embryology Bill. Two issues surrounding gender and mothering and parenting have stood out and provoked intense media interest. These are the retention of a duty to take account of the welfare of the child in providing fertility treatment and the proposed removal of the reference to 'the need for a father' as well as the change in the proposed Bill to recognise same-sex couples as legal parents of children conceived through the use of donated sperm, eggs or embryos.

Later female psychoanalysts challenged Freud's sexism and the influences of patriarchy to develop Freud's ideas. Their writings, stripped of Freud's patriarchal assumptions about the inferiority of femininity, are useful in understanding how sexual and gender identities develop (Sayers 1991). Examples include Deutsch (1944, 1945) who described for the first time the sexual development of girls, and Horney (1967) who described 'womb envy' in boys which, she argued, Freud had ignored due to his bias towards penis envy in girls. Both Deutsch and Horney analysed the interplay between interpersonal and patriarchal influences on sexual identity and gender development and intrapsychic conflicts during childhood and adolescence from a mother-centred approach rather than a father-centred one (Sayers 1991). Anna Freud modified Freud's child development theory to include the child's dependence on early mothering (Sayers 1991) while Klein (1975) rejected Freud's instinct theory of emotions in favour of a relational psychoanalysis based on the primary mothering relationship at the pre-Oedipal stage for both boys and girls. Sayers (1991) argues that this development from psycho-analysis' early father-centred, patriarchal beginnings to its current mother-centred focus has opened up the potential for utilising psychoanalytic theories within a feminist framework.

Psychoanalytic theories of sexual development emphasise the importance for both men and women of generative capability as part of gender identity (Raphael-Leff 1991; Pines 1993). Raphael-Leff (1991) has described the loss in infertility as generative death which means the loss of the individual's genes in future generations. Psychologically, Raphael-Leff (1991) and Pines (1993) argue that loss means the loss of psychological development which couples expect at an unconscious level but which is determined by the individual's psychological profile and personal history. Raphael-Leff (1991) and Pines (1993) also emphasise the influences of the social desirability of childbearing and parenting at a social and a psychological level. The necessity for society of the outcome of a child shapes the strength of the feeling society attributes to the loss infertile people feel. It may also influence the loss they are expected to express and indeed feel.

> **Reflection:**
>
> How far did your patient or couple reflect the ideas presented above about the importance of sexual development to later desire for children?

Gendered subjectivity and universal theories of caring: why do women care?

Gendered subjectivity

Chodorow (1974) argued that the cause of male dominance within patriarchy was based on how boys and girls learn to become gendered. She argued that boys learn through the Oedipus complex, experienced at the unconscious level through interiorised, subjective thoughts and feelings, to separate from their mother and identify with their fathers whose social roles are quite distinct. According to Chodorow (1974), through their inter-subjective and primary relationships boys develop a strong superego with a sense of autonomy as a separate adult. Girls identify with their mothers and through strong links with them, learn to become dependent, with a weaker superego or a less developed sense of autonomy, focusing on relationships in adult life rather than independent action. Again, they achieve this through the experience of internal, subjective and unconscious thoughts and feelings interacting with inter-subjective feelings from their primary relationships. The girl learns through her experience of being mothered to become a mother and is identified as such by society. The boy on the other hand does not learn to relate to others in the same way and becomes more focused on matters outside the family. Thus social relations between men and women shape the psychological attributes of gendered subjectivity learnt by girls and boys through the social construction of mothering and fathering played out in the Oedipus complex and separation from mother. Subjectivity includes social identity as well as the meanings individuals and society place on gender; gendered subjectivity is often referred to as masculinity or femininity but it is always a tension between the individual experience of being masculine, his early experiences of learning masculinity and society's expectations of masculine behaviour and roles. An example of gendered subjectivities are the expectations patients in study 1 had about who they expected to care for them and why. Largely, they expected nurses to be female, mothers, and to be concerned with caring. Whereas they expected doctors to be less focused on caring and more concerned with the science and medicine behind their treatment cycle. In other words, their own personal gendered subjectivities shaped their expectations of female nursing roles.

Chodorow's later work (1989) emphasises that social relations are important in gendered subjectivity but places greater emphasis on psychology as a constitutive and determinative feature of human life than in previous work. She describes this process of the acquisition of gendered subjectivity as 'a multiplex account of the dynamics of gender, sexuality, sexual inequality and domination' (1989:5) which is affected by the individual's psychic life and primary relationships.

Gilligan (1982; 1993) again drawing on psychoanalytic theories, used a psychological developmental process to argue that women are more focused than men on relationships and connectedness which is expressed as caring. This process is shaped by patriarchal social relations and male dominance during childhood which require men to be independent and women to be dependent adults. Patriarchal relations between men and women are reproduced as boys separate from their mothers and learn to separate from others, and girls remain connected to their mothers and consequently learn to be connected in their social relationships.

There are different interpretations of the extent to which Gilligan argues whether the association between women and caring is an empirical observation rather than a biological given, notably Harbison (1992) and Davies (1995). My reading of her work is that it is unclear how far she thinks that caring and connectedness is a female characteristic and how far it may be a question of the lack of voice for male caring and connectedness. Indeed, she explicitly does not address this issue: *'When I hear my work being cast in terms of whether women and men are really (essentially) different, or who is better than whom, I know I have lost my voice, because these are not my questions. .....And, my questions are about psychological processes and theory, particularly theories in which men's experience stands for all of human experience – theories which eclipse the lives of women and shut out women's voices'* (1993:xiii).

Conclusions

Chodorow (1989:167) argues that it is this concern with the social and the *intrapsychic* which is the potential contribution of feminist psychoanalysis for feminist social theory. I would argue that Chodorow's insight here is useful for fertility nurses either as women or men and suggest considering the following points before you go on to read the next chapter:

- Think about how infertile patients' experiences of infertility are shaped by their gendered development earlier in their lives and how their gendered development shapes their expectations of their future roles as parents. Gendered subjectivity and development explain why infertility is so emotionally powerful – it effects individuals' expectations of their future lives, their gendered identities and the meaning they give to being men and women. On top of that, infertility has a personal and a social effect – it affects internal feelings as well as social experiences.

- Think about how nurses' own internal feelings are affected when confronted with their patients' infertility – what feelings does their caring for infertile women raise about their own fertility? How are their experiences of parenting and fertility influential in shaping their attitudes towards infertile people's experiences?

- Think about how nurses' personal gendered subjectivities affect their relationships with infertile women and men? Do they expect certain masculine and feminine behaviours in infertile men and women? Do they expect certain mothering and fathering behaviours even in infertile women?

- Think about how nurses, especially female nurses, may reinforce expectations for female patients that their yearning for motherhood can be fulfilled through ARTs or only through ARTs?

In the next chapter I will present some data from study 1 which links the arguments I have made in Chapters 2 and 3 around the nature of caring and the role emotions play in shaping the nurse–patient relationship.

Part II

Caring and the experience of infertility

Chapter 4
The nature of caring and managing emotions in fertility nursing[10]

In Chapter 2, I outlined the theoretical background to caring and emotions in this book; in Chapter 3, I have provided an overview of the experience of infertility from psychological and psychoanalytic perspectives. I concluded with a description of a framework for understanding fertility nursing and fertility nurse–patient relationships (the acquisition of gendered subjectivity). In this chapter, I draw on some data from study 1 to illustrate this framework and discuss the nature of caring and the role of emotions in fertility nursing.

The main findings from study 1 were that patients described caring relationships with nurses as largely practical; the nursing role was described as 'being there' in the clinic and 'hovering' in order to be useful when necessary to patients and doctors. Patients also suggested that having female nurses supporting them during their time in the clinics was important, i.e. being a woman was important to being a nurse. Patients did not describe their relationships with nurses as being intimate or emotionally close, rather they sensed an emotional awareness which included an emotional distance which they were happy with. I argue that these forms of emotional awareness and distance mean that nurses were 'good enough' in the sense that they provided what the patients needed. As a result of managing emotions in this way, the nurses' main role was to run the clinics, support the doctors and guide patients through their clinic visits.

In the following chapters, I present data from two empirical studies. At the end of each chapter I will suggest reflections on the

---

[10] This chapter is developed from ideas previously published in: Allan, H. T. (2001) A 'good enough' nurse: supporting patients in a fertility unit. *Human Fertility* **4**: 18–23; Allan, H. T. (2002) Nursing the clinic, being there and hovering: ways of caring in a British fertility unit. *Journal Advanced Nursing*, **38**(1):86–93.

particular material presented in each chapter. However, you might also like to make a note of your reactions to the data I present within each chapter and consider:

How far are these data relevant and transferable to where you work?

Patients' descriptions of caring: a practical activity

Patients' descriptions of caring

According to patients, caring included features that have been previously identified in the literature as central to person-centred caring (Ersser 1997). They spoke, for example, of nurses' communication skills, nurses being calm and reaching out to the patient, talking to the patient, being encouraging, being knowledgeable, and using teaching skills. Louise sums up many of these attributes by saying that caring was having time to ask questions:

> It's just someone who understands, who knows the fact that when you're here, you've got so much time ... you feel that you can ask questions you really want to ask. And here you can sit there, and have it explained. And if you don't understand, you can have it explained again.

More generally, women commonly described caring as a 'being there', as Rebecca says:

> Being in the background. They're by my side and just asking if I'm alright.

Physical comfort and efficiency, while assisting with a procedure, were also described as part of caring by patients, which research on physical caring by Gardner and Wheeler (1981, 1987), Van Essen and Sjoden (1991) also suggests. Physical comfort, according to patients, could vary from 'being there' to giving a caring pat or talking a patient through a procedure. This emphasis on physical caring was observed during participant observation. The most obvious form of caring was physical, as this example from my observation notes shows:

Observing an intrauterine insemination in room 2. Maria assisting doctor. She touched, talked and joked with the woman. When the cervix was gripped with forceps (posterior) Maria said *'Well done, well done...nearly done'*, etc. Just touched her, with her hand on her shoulder, didn't stroke her. Very calm and soft tones. Doctor didn't interfere. Doctor told woman exactly what was happening. Both seemed to put her at ease very skillfully. Maria also was very efficient with the trolley, pack and procedure. Quite direct with her instructions to the woman. Also direct with her movements – purposeful.

Physical care here is demonstrated by Maria's touch, her use of voice and tone, her use of humour, and the way she acknowledged that the patient may feel pain when the cervix was gripped. Caring was also shown by the technical expertise with which Maria assisted and cleared away the medical equipment. The nurse physically cared for the patient without engaging in a close emotional or intimate relationship with her.

While patients were aware that nurses assisted doctors, and clearly differentiated between doctors' and nurses' roles, they also described the nursing role as being to support the doctors, with the nurse being the practical person who organised things and ran the clinics. Sarah described nurses as:

> *Being concerned with the longer term type of care ... the before and after.*

Nilima thought nurses were *'go-betweens'* while Tracey emphasised that doctors did not explain, or did not do so in terms patients understood, whereas nurses *'explain things in simpler terms I may understand'*. Nurses were also more approachable. As Sonya described, nurses *'can be asked silly questions'* and Louise said that *'asking them questions will not be a waste of their time'*. Finally, patients felt that, because nurses were more organised and were present all the time, they had the knowledge and authority to run things.

Patients' descriptions of their relationships with nurses involved some degree of emotional awareness on the nurse's part, and their descriptions of caring describe nurses as 'being there' to respond if needed, as Davies (1995) also contends. Patients also described nurses' ability to communicate as being characterised by being truthful, demonstrating concern and dealing with each person as an individual, which Bowden (1995), among others, describes as ethical caring. Both being there and caring ethically are skilled activities which do not need to be based on close emotional relationships. As Savage (1995:124) has argued, 'closeness' enacted through physical and emotional intimacy in nurse–patient relationships is not necessarily emotionally intense. Patients in this study described their relationships with nurses as close but not emotionally intense; for example, they often did not know nurses' names or any personal details. The nurse–patient relationship was based on social acquaintance rather than physical or emotional intimacy, although some degree of physical intimacy was required because of the nature of fertility treatments. This situation of enforced physical intimacy (see description of intrauterine insemination above) may, of course, have been why patients avoided emotional intimacy (as Savage 1995, found in another nursing context) and, indeed, some patients actively rejected emotional intimacy by maintaining distance from nurses in the clinics.

Reflection:

What have couples or women said to you about caring in the past? Have they valued caring and if so, how?

An emotional awareness

I have used the term 'emotional awareness' to describe this level of emotional support, which was not intense and did not involve emotional intimacy or closeness, but in which patients were aware of nurses' concern, as the examples above demonstrate. Patients did not always demand an emotional response but were aware that this was a possibility, and they described two aspects of emotional awareness in detail:

'knowing what I'm going through as a woman'

'being there in the background'

Being there as a woman

Most patients described nurses as mother figures who were aware

The nature of caring and managing emotions

of what they were going through; they frequently referred positively to nurses either being mothers or women. For example, Rebecca said:

Women may be more understanding than men. Being a female nurse, they've either had children or they've had this procedure, they've seen the good and bad of it all, they've had the experience of it all.

Susan was even more emphatic:

It's important to have a female nurse. I don't even tell my mother about these problems...they're older and I can approach them. They know what I'm going through because they've got the experience. Obviously, I don't know if they've got children but they've seen it, rather than a younger nurse coming here...you know, she might think, 'I don't want children. What's your problem?' sort of thing.

Other patients were clear that they preferred female nurses:

I don't think I'd like a male nurse. That's not being sexist or nothing but I don't think I would. (Tracey)

It's all about the caring role and I'm sure a man could do it as well. But ... you can accept a male doctor but not a male nurse. We are different (men and women). (Rebecca)

While patients described nurses as mothers and women and associated caring with being a woman and understanding their situation, gender was used in a different way when referring to doctors. Tracey suggested that if a doctor were female, she would be able to understand her patients' needs and communicate effectively:

The doctor was a woman (to do the X-ray) and she was far better at communicating to me what she was doing ... from my point of view, I feel more comfortable with women.

Dawn more clearly states that male doctors cannot understand her experiences because of their gender:

I don't care how much experience Dr X has, he's not a woman is he?

Although gender was important for patients, as these quotes show, some felt a doctor's personality and general approach could overcome issues around gender and intimate examinations:

> *Dr – is very nice. I must admit when I first saw him, I said to my husband, 'I'm not letting him examine me'. He has been very nice and gentle … you build a relationship with your doctor as time goes on* (Sonya).

While these data suggest that gender influences how both female nurses and male and female doctors are perceived, there are two interesting omissions. None of the patients suggested that female doctors cared in the same way as nurses, despite their shared gender. Neither did patients comment on the potential role of male nurses in caring.

Being there in the background and hovering

'Being there in the background' during physical examinations and in the clinics was a second feature of emotional awareness. Sarah described this as 'an awareness that someone understands'. The term emotional awareness therefore seemed an appropriate description for something which is low key, can vary from a physical action to an emotional response and may be never more than a possibility. Patients emphasised that the support offered by nurses in the corridor was a positive feature of the clinic because it offered a way of 'being there'.

'Being there' was a term also used by staff to describe the nursing role in this clinic. It included a familiarity with and knowledge of patients' needs and being there to run the clinic. Nurses appeared to manage being there by an activity I called 'hovering'.

When I first observed Phoebe, one of the specialist nurses, assisting Shula's (a registrar) medical consultations, I wondered if she became bored because she just seemed to 'hover' and 'do nothing' – these are terms I used in my observation notes. Then I realised that she was hovering with a purpose, which was to intervene if the situation demanded.

I observed that Phoebe would hover and sometimes intervene either to support Shula or the patient. Sometimes, she would intervene physically to support the patient (by holding an arm, writing a form) and she would always go out with the patient to see her out of the clinic and use this opportunity to ask if there was anything she needed to ask. As there was no receptionist in

The nature of caring and managing emotions

for some clinics, Phoebe and Shirley, both specialist nurses, arranged appointments and scans and dealt with telephone queries and medical records. Their involvement at all these levels offered a range of possibilities of interacting with patients from an informed position, and to answer questions not asked or missed during the medical interview.

Another description of hovering is given by Lizzie and Suki, two of the gynaecology nurses working in the AR clinics, who said that being there involved being in the corridor, usually doing something which could be left or waiting for something to do. This presence meant that they were visible to patients and waiting passively to act or ready to respond. Hovering with the intention to respond to patient need was a strong feature of the nursing work in the clinics.

The following extract from an observation in the scanning room is an example of the different ways of hovering:

> South American woman – no involvement from Alicia, doctor on his own. It appears Alicia has not 'acted' but she has been there to respond to demand. She got the table ready, prepared the environment, stayed in the background if needed. (A)

> Next patient, Indian woman – positive pregnancy test and scan. Very modest woman who did not speak or did not understand English – her husband translated for her. They seemed to have their own explanations for what was going on but the doctor didn't try to incorporate these into the meaning of the scan. Alicia responded to this woman's modesty positively and tried her best to keep her covered while the doctor tried to scan her which was actually difficult as she didn't want her skirt drawstring undone. Alicia touched her and spoke kindly to her – lowered voice. (B)

I considered that Alicia, a health care assistant (HCA), performed a skilled activity in (A) and (B). Being there could be passive (A) or active (B) according to when the nurse felt she was needed – leaving the doctor to interact with a patient but ready to intervene if necessary. The nurse needed to be there physically to be able to 'hover', actively or passively to 'be there'.

Managing intimacy and emotions

Justifying being there

Justifying being there

The caring activities performed by nurses that I have described were under threat from suggestions to devolve some nursing tasks to health care assistants (HCAs) – a general trend in nursing in the UK (Clifford 1995, Warr 1998). I discuss this in more detail in Chapter 8. The pressure on managers to justify activity which was not visible or recorded (see also McKenna 1995) led them to argue that unqualified staff should undertake activities such as 'being there'. Sharma, the gynaecology nursing manager, thought a relative could replace a trained nurse 'just' to give support during an emotional time:

> *You don't need a trained nurse to give TLC (tender loving care).*

While nursing staff defended the concept of 'being there' as a nursing activity, they were aware that this was difficult to justify to managers as it appeared invisible, and there was tension during the participant observation period between nurses and their managers. This misunderstanding was not resolved until Alicia, the HCA who staffed the scanning room, missed the implications of a woman's set of observations one day. This situation resolved managers' reluctance to allow trained nurses to assist doctors in clinics, as nursing staff were able to argue that a trained nurse, even if they were 'just' assisting the doctor, was necessary in case her nursing skills were required. 'Being there', according to them, was having the knowledge to act should the patient or situation demand it. The HCA could not do this because her knowledge and ability to negotiate were not sufficient in this case.

In the normal routine of the clinics, nursing work went unrecorded and only became visible when an emergency arose. Phoebe, a specialist nurse, gave a good example of how difficult it was to record what she did and thereby justify her role:

> P: *Really you're talking about self-auditing, aren't you? Writing down, well, 'I did this', 'I did that' and 'I measured that'. That's very difficult.*
> HA: *Where would you do it? Would you do it in the medical notes?*
> P: *Um, yes in the medical notes. But it would just be an annotation really. So you might, say if you'd had a really heavy session on the telephone, you might write 'long chat' in the*

notes. And the gist of what that's about. I don't capture what it is I do on paper. And I can't. I find it difficult to put into words … but I am quite confident of my value in this clinic.

Perhaps because of this invisibility, nursing work was not evident and nurses felt under pressure to change their role – to make it more visible. They felt under pressure to justify a qualified nursing presence in the clinics and specific roles such as chaperoning and admitting patients. This pressure was made worse by developments in other AR clinics which they either felt untrained for or felt would diminish their caring role in chaperoning and being in the clinic to support the doctors. For example, one doctor proposed at a staff meeting that receptionists could answer the phone to release nurses in the clinic for nursing duties. He felt that nurses could be used to cover routine, medical tasks supervised by the clinic doctor, while the receptionist did the non-nursing work, such as phone work and admissions (including blood pressures). This was exactly the nursing work that was valued by patients and could also be life-saving, as the nurses argued. The skills and knowledge required to be there emerged as I spent longer in the field. The term used by participants to describe these nursing skills was 'running the clinics'.

Being there to run the clinic: 'she gets all my bits and pieces together'

Being there to run the clinic

Running the clinics was a key role in the two AR clinics and one described in detail by nursing and non-nursing staff. Of course, to run the clinic the nurse needed to be there, so being there to 'fix things up' emerged as another feature of the nurse's role and further emphasised the practical nature of caring in the clinics.

Patients described their reliance on nurses to guide them through their clinic visits and to direct them between departments during the same visit. Lizzie, one of the gynaecology nurses, explained how she directed patients through the confusing situation:

When the patient first comes, they meet us and you sort of build up a relationship with them, which is nice. And I suppose all the instructions and everything that the doctors do not have time to go into fully is up to you; and all the forms when they're unsure of things is left up to you. So yes, the nurse is in the middle, directing all.

The picture Lizzie conveyed was reinforced through participant observation as I observed nurses taking over control of patients' movements within the clinic; directing them to the waiting room, summoning them to the doctor's consultation room, directing them elsewhere or giving them instructions prior to leaving the clinic.

This picture of nurses being there as a physical presence, a safety barrier or a familiar figure, was a key feature of descriptions of the nursing role in the clinic. Patients described nurses' presence at the beginning of the clinic as 'easing in':

They're the key point ... They're the first you know and they kind of ease people in.

Easing people into the clinic, sorting out problems and dealing with patients personally was a way of introducing or welcoming them to the clinic before the main interview with a doctor. Easing in could be seen as a way of 'nursing the clinic' by easing patients into a way of behaving in order that they would not be a problem in the consulting room, for example, by needing an X-ray report or not being ready for an intrauterine insemination.

After the clinic was all over at the end of a clinic, calm descended after the emotion of the session. Staff remarked that they felt they worked in a chaotic atmosphere at times. The nurse was described as the lynchpin by medical and reception staff. Doctors commented that, without the nurse being 'visible' in the corridor, they felt lost. They would sometimes wander around looking for a clinic nurse, unable to proceed with the routine of the clinic unless reassured by the presence of a nurse to direct patients out of the consulting room or find an appropriate form to request an investigation.

Staff perceptions of chaos were different to patients' descriptions of the clinics, which were that it was busy and confusing rather than chaotic. It may be that the patients' perceptions were restricted to a personal rather than a holistic view. Patients were not caught up in the drama as staff were. If patients left feeling that their needs were attended to, then the clinic continued without them and they remained largely untouched by the chaos. Patients essentially seemed more interested in the outcome – a baby – and in their progress towards this through the clinic rather than the process when in the clinic, as Gorovitz (1994) suggests. Their priorities were focused on managing their infertility and they did not get embroiled in busy clinics.

The nurse's role in coordinating the action in the middle of a busy clinic was difficult to identify. When I asked Lizzie, a gynaecology nurse, to describe what she did, she said:

> L: *A general pair of hands to help with everything ... which I don't really mind. It's got to be done. The remark 'That's not my job' hasn't really come into it ... the way I've been trained that doesn't really come into it.*
> HA: *What?*
> L: *It's not my job and this, that and the other. It doesn't matter. It has to be done and you get on and do it.*

I felt that the implication of Lizzie's phrase, 'that's not my job', summed up the nurses' role in running the clinics, which was to be a flexible response to a range of demands, such as searching for results, booking appointments or ordering drugs, taking patients for scans, supporting distressed patients, and answering telephone enquiries. Lizzie was aware that responsibility for the running of the clinic and the return to calm afterwards, was the nurses'. They would do whatever was demanded of them to achieve closure or 'end of the clinic' in their words, although many of the tasks were not seen as nursing by managers.

The nurses' role was, therefore, management of the process in time and space as well as management of emotions.

The nursing role was shaped through the needs of the clinic at a practical level: 'nursing the clinic' and through responding to patient demand, 'being there' in the clinic as a resource, a problem solver or support. As Roberta, a patient, described: 'getting all my bits and pieces together'. By which she meant having her scans arranged, her drugs written up and her next appointment arranged.

The physical presence of nurses also meant that doctors felt a familiarity too, and they referred to nurses being present in the clinic for different reasons. They emphasised the continuity of the nurse in the clinic, which extended her knowledge of the specialty and established good working relationships with doctors. Although doctors emphasised the importance of nurses being there, they focused on them being there to facilitate the medical work.

Acknowledging this difference between the importance of caring for patients and supporting medical staff is not new (Street 1992). However, the doctors' behaviour and attitudes in shaping the nursing role in the clinics were important, as they shaped the 'nursing of the clinic and the doctor' rather than 'nursing the patient'.

Personal qualities

Personal qualities

Participants considered nurses' personal qualities to be the defining feature of nursing which enabled them to assist doctors and help patients, as one patient's description suggested: 'Sister will see you now'. These traditional roles and attributes confirm previous research (Hughes *et al.* 1958, Anderson 1973, Smith 1992) but are perhaps surprising in view of the emergence of 'new' nursing (Savage 1995), advanced and specialist nursing and target driven organisational reform. Nurses in the clinic described nurses needing to be patient, fun, on an even keel, empathic, approachable, warm, well-controlled, non-threatening, encouraging and mature enough to know their own values. Receptionists thought nurses should be caring, able to give 100% to patients and sympathetic.

Doctors described nurses as being able to communicate, being female, caring, able to bond with people, friendly, human, responsible and calming; however, they also said that nurses should be knowledgeable. Although, one consultant suggested that:

> In an appointment like that (of a fertility nurse) I would put the emphasis on the communication skills rather than the technical aspects because those can be cultivated.

His views are interesting because, although Phoebe ran one of his clinics as a specialist nurse largely on her own, he emphasised the personal skills rather than the technical. As Phoebe said:

> Nurses can act as a safety buffer between patient and doctor, they are less threatening than doctors and can interpret the doctors' language. They fulfill a patient's psychological need.

The nature of caring and managing emotions

None of the staff described a nurse as an independent practitioner with specific skills but rather as a caring human being. Lizzie, a gynaecology nurse, was even more down to earth and succinctly described her role:

a general pair of hands helping with everything.

> **To summarise this section:**
> - I have suggested that the nursing role was essentially practical and concerned with running the clinic and managing a busy, at times chaotic atmosphere
> - being a woman as a nurse was considered important to patients
> - being present in the clinic through activities such as being there, running the clinic and hovering, nurses supported both patients and doctors
> - through being there, nurses were able to provide an emotional awareness which patients noticed, even if this emotional awareness did not result in close or intimate relationships
> - at times, emotional distance was the more commonly observed emotional behaviour in the clinic.

Observations of non-caring: emotional distance

Observations of non-caring

I use the term 'non-caring' to describe nurses acting practically for patients while at the same time maintaining an emotional distance from them when patients became emotional. In contrast to observations of emotional awareness when the nurse appeared to react or respond to a patient's need (often non-verbal need), emotional distance occurred when the patient showed emotional distress in the presence of a nurse, but it was not acknowledged. Observed instances of emotional distance which occurred frequently was when a nurse hovered in the corridor of the clinic waiting for a patient to emerge from a medical consultation. On emerging, patients would be ushered by the nurse to the receptionist or the pharmacy. At these times, patients might sometimes appear reluctant to leave the clinic, hang around the nurses' desk and show clear signs of anxiety or distress which would be ignored by the nurse who would be running the clinic. An example of this type of emotional distance or non-caring occurred when Evelyn, having spent 5 minutes arranging the next set of appointments with an overtly anxious patient, literally turned her back and started sorting patient notes, thereby ignoring the patient until the latter very slowly left the clinic. By overtly anxious behaviours, I observed the patient asking anxious questions, toying incessantly with her diary, making self-deprecating remarks about how unsuccessful she was likely to be during her present cycle and literally taking 5 minutes to walk away down the corridor to leave the clinic.

Managing emotions, managing the clinic

Non-caring could also arise when patients would be taken into the sister's room for information on the next stage of their investigations. These information sessions lasted on average 5–10 minutes and were primarily concerned with the transfer of relevant information. Any opportunities for caring and sharing of anxieties were dependent on the nurse's responsibilities in running the clinics. The door to the room was left ajar so the nurse could continue to respond to situations arising in the clinic and for other staff to use the room. In these instances, non-caring was the management of the nurse–patient interaction so that emotions could not be shared. Non-caring was therefore both the management of emotions in order that they did not interrupt the clinic and the lack of response to emotions. It was a complex activity occurring regularly during a clinic alongside caring. The ability to combine caring and non-caring was achieved through an activity I have described as 'nursing the clinic' where the clinic and the doctor became the focus of nursing rather than the patient. In a bizarre way then, 'nursing the clinic' met both patient and staff expectations of the practical nature of the nursing role as described above.

'Nursing the clinic and the doctor' was evident in the following excerpt from my field notes where the nurses, Evelyn and Suki, were aware of the patient's potential distress but acted to avoid any involvement.

> USS comes back from the dept with Joanna's pictures. Goes into Dr Thomas. Suki knows this is about Joanna's follicles

which are too many and there aren't any dominant ones. Suki says to me *'She will be upset. It's such a shame'* and shakes her head. *'It's such a shame to abandon the cycle. All that hope'.* So, she knows about Joanna's results and is concerned and aware that she will be upset. When Joanna arrives, Evelyn (who has been told about the USS result) ignores Joanna after a brief hello in the public waiting room. Joanna is upset and starts to cry; it is unclear whether she knows the result but clearly has found the scan and the wait to see Dr Thomas distressing. Evelyn places Joanna in the waiting room, a public space, to cry but ignores her emotion. The clinic goes on with seeing patients.

Dr Graham calls her next patient. Dr Thomas rings and Evelyn calls Joanna. Evelyn walks with Joanna from the waiting room to the consulting room but fails to acknowledge her pain and loss even though she is aware of it.

Joanna sees Dr Thomas on her own and hears the results of the scan without a nurse being present. Evelyn comes out of the consulting room after showing Joanna into Dr Thomas and says to Suki *'She's very upset, Joanna. If you want to help me, come and get the cake'.* There is someone leaving today, one of the clerks, and Evelyn has made a cake for tea.

In this excerpt, Suki and Evelyn 'nursed the clinic' as they welcomed the patients, showed them into the consulting rooms and responded to doctors' demands. But they did not 'nurse' Joanna. It was not possible to know whether Joanna felt she was being ignored and my interpretation of non-caring raises interesting questions about what ethical justification there can be for emotional distance in the face of evident distress such as crying. In interviews, nurses described their non-intimacy as a necessary basis for caring and did not comment on the ethical questions that non-caring raised for me. It also calls into question the ethic of caring outlined in Chapter 2 where theorists, such as Benner & Wrubel (1989), assume that nurses care towards and about their patients. Clearly in this instance and others I observed, nurses cared about but did not care towards – in fact, they were non-caring. Rather than seeing this episode as an ethical dilemma where they did not care, on questioning at the subsequent tea party, the nurses explained that they understood it as being a private issue to do with Joanna's upset and distress.

Running the clinic

Another way given to explain the non-caring behaviours was by seeing the nurses' time as constrained by paperwork and running the clinics, i.e. about fair distribution of resources where both nurses and patients understood the nurses to be caring within the constraints of time and resources. One patient described this by saying,

> *If I were in that position I would be thinking, 'Well, if I could get this paper work done I could go home on time instead of sitting chatting to someone.'*

Nurses engaged in activities like 'nursing the clinic and doctor', which were non-caring, while at the same time describing in interviews that they cared and had close relationships with particular patients. Suki and Evelyn were aware of Joanna's upset and were not uncaring. They cared about Joanna as is evident in Suki's comments but chose not to care for her emotionally at that moment. Instead, they engaged in non-caring activities such as running the clinic and ensuring Joanna was seen as quickly as possible. By understanding this behaviour from a psychoanalytic perspective, I was led by the data to consider the emotions rather than the ethics of the situation from a rational standpoint (Fabricius 1991a).

In interviews, staff described nurses being more concerned with caring to complement the medical work doctors undertook. In contrast to these descriptions of close, caring relationships, as the above excerpt shows, I did not observe emotional involvement but rather an avoidance of emotional contact, which I called 'non-caring' or emotional distance. One interpretation of this emotional distance could be that nurses were constrained to 'nurse the clinic and the doctor' by their oppressive position vis-à-vis doctors (Gamarnikov 1978). In psychoanalytic interpretations of organisations and emotions, there is a tension between how much behaviour results from individual psychology and how much is the result of organisational practices (Menzies 1970; Obholzer & Zagier Roberts 1994). I argue that the nurses' behaviours around caring and non-caring were mutually shaped by the organisation and by their personal defenses against anxiety. To locate the origins in either one or the other can move away from constructive dialogue as I believe has happened in the literature on emotions and caring.

The nature of caring and managing emotions

My thoughts about 'non-caring' and the presence of emotional distance in the nurse–patient relationship were triggered by the patients' interviews. Patients described a discrepancy between what they said they wanted, practical caring, emotional awareness, and the types of relationships they developed with nurses, which I have described as emotionally distant. Patients described nurses as caring and supportive while, at the same time, also as strangers, as the following quotes show:

> I don't know her name. I don't know whether she's been here for the last year or not. There are people wandering through the room and I've never really known who they are. (Sonya)

Patients also expressed anger toward staff, including nurses, for ignoring their anxieties, which seemed to be inconsistent with their descriptions of nurses understanding their position as women:

> My overriding frustration must be when you are sitting there with a live specimen for over two hours and you think 'why?' because the person who's just come for a consultation should be seen after the patients with live specimens. Why is it so important to make love within the last 18 hours if you're going to keep me waiting after that time here? (Roberta)

These descriptions of the reality of being cared for were contradictory strands in the data. They suggested that there might have been a reluctance to acknowledge that caring was not possible all the time even though the patients were aware that nurses cared about them. I have interpreted this data by arguing that the nurses remained 'good enough' by offering an emotional awareness and an emotional distance which was all that was possible within the constraints of their ability to care, and the time and resources available for care.

Despite these constraints, patients were tolerant toward the nurses' non-caring behaviours and positive in their descriptions of caring such as being there as a woman, emotional awareness as well as the practical information and support they believed they received. I argue that their management of their own infertility was complemented by the nurses' caring and non-caring behaviours and was overall, despite some anxiety and anger, 'good enough'.

Managing intimacy and emotions

The 'good enough' nurse

The 'good enough' nurse

Patients' and nurses' descriptions of their relationships seemed at times too positive, even unreal to me. Patients' descriptions of the nurses they wanted were fantasies of a nurse who was an ideal as Muff (1982) also argues. This fantasy nurse seemed to coexist with the real nurse who was 'good enough' in patients' accounts, able to 'be there' in the background and convey an emotional awareness while, at the same time, able to focus on the practicalities of running an AR clinic, 'getting my bits and pieces'. The fantasy nurse patients described was giving, caring, motherly and warm and the real nurse was there if needed, emotionally aware but not intimate. Like the ideal mother and the good enough mother, patients constructed the 'ideal' nurse, while the reality was 'good enough' (Fabricius 1991a).

Fabricius (1991a) suggests that patients emotionally want the ideal nurse who can mother them because they regress and become dependent when ill. However, the good enough nurse is sufficient because, in reality, patients are able to cope with that dependency on their own without regressing far enough to need a mothering figure. Fabricius (1991a) argues that the good enough nurse is able to tolerate demands on herself to retreat from emotional engagement or awareness if she feels overwhelmed. It is this retreat from engagement, which I argue is the non-caring observed in this study.

Knowing your patient

The 'knowing' described by patients and nurses was more accurately an ideal knowing based on nurses' occupational position and being a woman rather than knowing from her real relationships with the nurses in the clinics. As Tracey, a patient, described it:

> Doctors do not talk to patients, doctors go straight to the point … say what they have to say and then you're out … they think that's the nurse's role don't they? They're here to treat the patient basically, they're not listening. Not to console them or…

Tracey criticised the doctors for not 'consoling' her, but did not appear to have been consoled by the nurses. She was not intimate with the nurses, as she said:

The nature of caring and managing emotions

I just ask them [nurses] how they are. I don't really know them.

The nurses did not generally accompany her into the doctor's room and did not know what happened in her consultations. She had no opportunity to be intimate as she had no contact other than social contact with the nurses. She split the nurses and doctors, the doctors were bad and the nurses were good. But this was an idealised version of reality, the fantasy nurse rather than the real nurse she met in the clinic. The discrepancy between the fantasy and the real nurse emerged as patients described their expectations of caring. Patients expressed their anxieties which were emotional and distressing. When I asked if they had told their concerns to the staff, they said they had not for a variety of reasons. Some said they felt it was not appropriate; some had not had the opportunity; and some did not wish to. In this way, 'non-caring' was mutually shaped by patients' and nurses' opportunities and abilities to cope with emotional involvement. Intimacy and distance created a tension in the spaces of the clinics where nursing took place.

Patient initiated relationships

This is not to deny the descriptions of the 'close' relationships described by nurses in the data. However, it does suggest that these relationships happened, at times, as a result of patient action rather than being initiated by nurses. In most interactions with patients, either the doctor was there and the nurse could not act independently unless she chose to do so afterwards, or the nurse was not there to witness the doctor–patient interaction and the nurse was acting in the dark. Therefore, the lack of space and time available meant that patients, while aware of nurses' potential emotional awareness, realised the capacity for emotional involvement was constrained by space, privacy and time. In addition, nurse-led behaviour, such as 'nursing the clinic and the doctor', prevented nursing the patient. The nurse–patient relationship appeared to be shaped at the same time by the doctor–nurse relationship rather than a response to patient need and by a belief that emotional intimacy was inappropriate in a nurse–patient relationship. Shirley, one of the specialist nurses, was, potentially, the obvious exception to this analysis as she saw patients on her own and did have the opportunity to 'nurse the patient'. However, she also managed emotions by an emotional distance. It appeared that even when barriers to emotional distance were removed, nurses did not engage in emotionally close relationships.

There seemed a contradiction between patients saying they valued the nurses' being there and their personalities on the one hand, and patients not wanting to communicate openly about their concerns with nurses. Patients did not express their needs and managed their infertility and being a patient privately. I suggest that the 'good enough' nurse was the emotionally aware nurse who could intervene if necessary. The ideal or fantasy nurse was the nurse many patients described as a good nurse but whom they did not need as they actively managed their own emotions. The nurses' behaviours also influenced patients. The interview data with patients showed an awareness of nurses' busy work, the appropriateness of seeking support and their own responsibilities, as well as their need to remain in control.

Additionally, patients had their own expectations of appropriate patient behaviour. In these ways they contributed to the 'good enough' nurse in Fabricius' (1991b) terms by 'holding' their emotions in check and by being independent when it was appropriate.

Nurses described a lack of closeness as a necessary feature of the nurse–patient relationship. While they described caring in therapeutic terms as well as more conventional terms, the nurses believed that caring was a key nursing activity which encompassed support rather than a therapeutic relationship. This form of caring emerged as a claim to care with an awareness that they could only care practically if they did not become too close to patients. Purkiss (1996) argues that issues of right and wrong must be put aside to examine the realities of caring. This raises ethical questions around whether it is possible to ignore an ethic of care or notions of justice in caring. I argue that by seeing caring and non-caring as a range of activities, which were possible psychoanalytically for nurses, I can understand how patients' and nurses' experiences of care were mutually constituted. I believe Purkis suggests an important way to put aside absolutes to consider how caring emerges from the realities of everyday practice which are framed by ethical questions, as well as how caring is framed as an absolute goal for nursing. This latter type of therapeutic caring remained an ideal, which the nurses struggled with when describing aspects of caring in their relationships with patients.

Discussion

I have argued that the data suggested that patients did not want emotional intimacy but valued the practical, everyday skills that nurses used to care. They also valued emotional awareness, which I have defined as a nurse's ability to convey, not always verbally, that a patient's concerns and anxieties have been understood. There was, however, a discrepancy between what patients said they wanted and what they received from nurses, even allowing for a desire for practical caring and emotional non-intimacy. This discrepancy occurred because nurses' priorities were to nurse the clinic and not the patient. This form of caring is not uncaring, but may provide a level of care in a space that allows patients to manage the social and medical experience of infertility.

> 'Nursing the clinic and the doctor', the way in which the nurses attended to the needs of the clinic and the doctor rather than of the patient, is a key finding for clinical nursing to emerge from this study.

This mode of nursing was achieved through being there, hovering and running the clinics. I have argued that these nursing activities are similar to and, at the same time, different from those previously described in the nursing literature, although Hunt and Meerabeau (1993) have also reported a lack of emotional expression in fertility and oncology clinics. These forms of caring are generally seen to be practical skills only, yet this study shows that the nurse has to combine emotional awareness to satisfy patient expectations and thus allow patients and nurses to 'hold' or manage emotions.

Caring and competence

Nurses also have to be knowledgeable to act when patients are at risk. Increasingly, these types of caring skills are being delegated to health care assistants, while nurses take on skilled medical tasks not only in fertility nursing, but in broader nursing contexts (Bradshaw 1995). The findings from this study, in particular, the subtlety involved in activities such as 'hovering', which offers an opportunity for emotional awareness, suggest that further erosion of the caring role of nurses, or extension of the traditional nursing role to include medical skills, may have detrimental effects on patient care and run counter to patient expectations. Daly & Carnwell (2003), in a recent discussion of the emergence of new nursing roles, suggest that nursing roles fall into three groups:

- **role extension** – whereby tasks from another profession are subsumed into nursing;

- **role expansion** – whereby the core elements of nursing are retained but the skills and knowledge become specialised;

- **role development** (**advanced roles**) – which incorporates extension and expansion but includes clinical autonomy to meet patient needs independently.

This data shows how in performing caring activities, nurses can observe and respond to patient need which might otherwise be missed by a less qualified health care worker.

In later chapters, I shall explore how taking on advanced roles which include medical tasks such as egg collection and embryo transfer, allow fertility nurses to provide continuity of care while at the same time developing and using expert knowledge and skills. As Barber *et al.* (1996) suggest, performing medical tasks in relationships where nurses know patients well may enhance embryo transfer rates; nurses performing embryo transfers potentially benefit the couple by offering continuity of care, which reduces stress and increases confidence. Data from this study suggests that these changes to fertility nurses' roles need to be evaluated further and, in particular, patients' opinions need to be sought. This data, if repeated in other fertility units, has implications for current government policies, which encourage and support the development of autonomous nursing practice (for certain levels of nurse) and the delegation of traditional nursing skills to health care assistants.

While the outpatient setting could be argued to have constrained the potential for developing the type of emotional relationship observed in inpatient settings (for example, Ersser 1997), the data suggested that neither nurses nor patients expected or valued intense emotional relationships. Could their expectations have been shaped by other considerations? Hunt & Meerabeau (1993) believe that consumerism may structure routinised and minimal interactions in the outpatient setting and this may influence patient expectations. Certainly, patients and staff were aware of how financial considerations influenced decision-making in fertility work. However, this awareness did not seem to affect the expectations that patients had of nurses or the type of caring in which it was appropriate for nurses to engage. I conclude that this emotional awareness is one form of caring, although other forms may be possible in outpatient settings and other patients may be more aware of more structural or financial constraints.

Caring theories have a common thread: they value care and seek to affirm caring values in a society where caring is the devalued, invisible work of women (Gilligan 1982, 1993; Hochschild 1995; Oakley 1993). To this end, the most popular caring theories in nursing have recently been located in the humanist tradition, which celebrates the potential for good in people (Uys 1980; Watson 1988; Meutzal 1988; Morse 1991). Humanism in nursing has emphasised that positive unconditional regard toward each person is the basis of human relationships which are equal and emotionally connected (Barber 1991; Ersser 1997). This is clearly expressed in Benner & Wrubel's (1989) popular theory of nursing which is based on an ethic of care.

The data in this study shows that nursing may include caring and non-caring behaviours, which meet patients' expectations of nursing as a practical, skilled activity which is not based on close, emotional involvement. Staff believed that these types of relationships prevented them from becoming too close to patients. The risks of potential closeness would only be greater if they formed closer relationships, as these quotes show from an informal conversation between myself, a nurse and a doctor:

> N: *I try not to get involved with them. And that's difficult because you see the same patient coming back month after month and you think 'oh I wish they'd get pregnant'. But um I try not to, I do think about it and that, but I try not to take it too much to heart. You know ... I'm not sure.*
> HA: *What would happen if you did take it to heart?*
> N: *I suppose I'd get upset because they're upset and worried and that and you take it all on. It can get a bit too much.* (Nurse)

Managing intimacy and emotions

I see 17 patients who are shattered and I come home and I'm shattered and that's three times a week. (Consultant)

None of the staff associated the emotional cost of caring and non-caring with their feelings of being 'shattered' and did not understand how supervision might be used to manage closer relationships with patients.[11] Following Menzies (1970) and later interpretations of her work (Fabricius 1991a, 1991b; Obholzer and Zagier Roberts 1994), I argue that caring, emotional awareness, and non-caring, emotional distance, may be necessary in psychoanalytic terms as defences against painful emotions in clinical practice.

Non-caring occurred when emotions were managed in particular ways in order to distance staff from patients. These defences may have been necessary psychically in order that the nurses could care practically for their patients. This way of working, combining caring and non-caring, conveyed a sense of emotional awareness (caring) which complemented the patients' desire for a 'good enough' caring which is achieved through the nurse 'being with' the patient to care when necessary.

One of the consequences of these types of nurse–patient relationships, which alternated between emotional awareness and distance, was a lack of articulation by patients of their emotional needs and recognition of these by staff. It was assumed that the 'ideal' nurse cared for patients' emotional needs at the same time as patients' needs were left unarticulated. Due to this assumption, there was confusion and uncertainty among nurses and doctors around the provision of therapeutic counselling in the unit and the boundaries between caring and counselling. In addition, staff believed that, while the relationships described in this paper as caring and non-caring were appropriate for most patients, there was also a need by some patients for a different type of relationship; more specifically, a counselling relationship.

Conclusion

An important implication from this study for clinical nursing is that traditional nursing skills used in 'being there' and 'hovering' are a skilled and valued aspect of patient care, experienced in a

---

[11] Supervision here refers to regular reflection on practice with a focus on the emotions raised through clinical interactions with patients.

relationship that is not always emotionally involved. I suggest that 'being there' is possible as a form of physical attendance that offers emotional awareness rather than emotional intimacy.

These findings call into question theories of nursing as therapy which promote a therapeutic relationship based on intimacy (Barber 1991; Ersser 1997). I argue that the types of less emotionally involved nurse–patient relationships described in this study, where caring is nevertheless experienced by patients, are valid ways of managing nurse–patient relations. I argue that less emotionally intense relationships may also be necessary as defences against painful emotions in clinical practice (Allan 2001).

Menzies (1970) argued a long time ago that nurses perform activities which are physically distasteful, distressing and frightening and which evoke painful feelings. To defend against the anxiety raised by these feelings, nurses in this study cared in ways which distanced themselves from patients in order to cope.

The data in study 1 suggested that this is both what patients expected and wanted from their relationships with nurses, a distance but at the same time an awareness that they cared. By caring in this way, nurses were able to get the work done and patients felt cared for. Fabricius (1991a) has argued that the ability to be 'good enough' is the quality nurses should strive for in their relationships with patients. If they are good enough, they can tolerate the pain they observe in patients at times and at other times withdraw when the pain gets too much and either refer on to other more appropriately qualified staff, such as fertility counsellors, or simply hand over to another nurse. Fertility counsellors in some units do offer support and supervision for clinical staff to help them cope with the emotions they meet in practice. If these nurses had been aware that they were caring (emotionally aware) and non-caring (emotionally distant), they may have been able to contain patients' feelings more consistently (by being caring) and referred Joanna and patients like her on to counselling support (by being able to recognise when they were being non-caring). Instead, such patients were left alone in their distress and their feelings denied while the illusion of the ideal nurse was maintained.

I have argued that this denial was partly contributed to by patients' expectations of nursing care which were to experience a level of emotional awareness, which would contribute to the management of their infertility. This emotional awareness was conveyed through traditional nursing skills such as chaperoning and being there.

I have acknowledged that ethical considerations can appear to be missing from a psychoanalytic interpretation of my data, which raises issues around how far nurses are personally responsible for caring and non-caring in the context of health care delivery in the NHS. For example, the nurses in this setting were not encouraged to recognise feelings arising from their interactions with patients and had not been offered clinical supervision by nursing management, unlike other staff elsewhere in the hospital. I am suggesting that a psychoanalytic interpretation of my data contributes to understanding the realities of care which include the pain of caring as well as the positive benefits of caring for patients and nurses. These nurses witnessed distress and alternated between caring and non-caring to tolerate being with patients. The idea of a 'good enough' nurse acknowledges the difficulties of caring and the necessity at times for non-caring, while contributing to the arguments for support for nurses doing the difficult work of nursing.

Reflection:

What conclusions do you draw about the nature of nurse–patient relationships after reading this chapter?
How far do you agree that nursing involves a degree of emotional distance in caring for patients?
Do you think chaperoning has a role in nursing today?

Chapter 5
Managing emotions and the body in fertility nursing: chaperoning brought up to date[12]

In this chapter, I draw on data from study 1 which describes women's experiences of the gendered body in AR clinics. I suggest that the concept of embodiment helps us to understand the effects of gender on the delivery of women's health services. The term chaperone is used to refer to accompanying a female patient by a female nurse (or healthcare assistant) during an intimate examination by a doctor (Whittaker 1993). I review the literature on gendered caring and the gendered role of nursing to suggest that the literature does not offer a way to understand women's preferences for female nurses as chaperones. I then review phenomenological approaches to embodiment, which may offer such an understanding.

The role of female nurse as chaperone may develop alternative understandings of nursing in this highly gendered field of practice. These understandings are potentially transgressive as they challenge currently accepted notions of professional development based on skills acquisition which are based on a mind–body split; they also appear to reinforce traditional gendered views of nursing.

Chaperoning

Chaperoning

The literature on chaperoning and the role of the female chaperone is limited. In the UK, writers are concerned with protecting doctors against litigation (RCOG 1997; Bignell 1999; Croft 1999; Torrance, Das & Allison 1999). The emphasis in these writings is on surveillance, the medico-legal consequences of non-chaperoning for the doctor–patient relationship and the

[12] Adapted from a previously published paper: Allan, H.T. (2005) Gender and embodiment in nursing: the role of the female chaperone in AR clinics *Nursing Enquiry* **12**(3): 175–183

practicalities of providing sufficient nurses to chaperone in busy gynaecology departments (Bignell 1999).

Whether nurses should chaperone, what chaperoning might mean to both patients and staff and what the consequences of chaperoning female patients are for male nurses or for male patients being cared for by female nurses are not explored in the literature (Editorial 2000; 2003). There are midwives who argue for women caring for women as birth attendants (Howell-White 1999; Lay 2000) but little attention has been given to the role of the female chaperone in the non-midwifery setting by feminists. Nor is heterosexuality challenged in these midwifery analyses. By this I mean that gender is assumed to be based on heteronormative assumptions around male and female genders, which fail to acknowledge the complexities of both individuals' experiences and responses to gender (Chodorow 1989; Davies 2003). The failure to address the cases of male patients being attended to by female nurses is an example of this heteronormative approach to gynaeco-logical and psychosexual examinations. In the small number of studies that explore men's experiences of illness in relation to the gendered role of nurses, it is suggested that male patients focus on the survival of their disease rather than relationships with nursing staff (Jones & Webb 1994). Although data on the effects of male nurses caring for male or female patients are limited, Miers (2000) argues that gay responses to HIV and AIDS may offer a potentially liberating way of exploring gender-sensitive care among networks of gay men that does not reinforce hegemonic masculinities.

More generally, social relations between men and women are shaped by the psychological attribute of gendered subjectivity (Chodorow 1989) [see Chapter 3] and, given that gender is a relational concept, shaped through interpersonal relationships and the environment (Davies 2003) as well as by psychological processes (Chodorow 1989). A shared gendered subjectivity, then, may offer one way of exploring the role of the female chaperone, particularly in the gendered field of reproductive technologies.

Gender and chaperoning

Central to ARTs are the gender roles of motherhood, fatherhood and parenthood (and the expressions of gendered subjectivity associated with each role), and the challenges these new reproductive technologies represent to traditional western values related to these gender roles (Cannell 1990). For example, motherhood is understood as being strongly linked with caring and emotional work (Gilligan 1982, 1993; Bowden 1997) as discussed in Chapter 2. This association between women and motherhood means that nurses became strongly linked with mothering and emotional work through the association between nursing, caring and women's work in the home during the nineteenth and twentieth centuries (Reverby 1987; Miers 2000). Davies (1995) argues that the gendered nature of caring in nursing is partly determined by its largely female workforce along with the context of health care in which nursing takes place. Nursing has a gendered position vis-à-vis medicine (Davies 1995; Porter 1995), which developed historically through the association of nursing with female domestic work (Reverby 1987; Kuhse 1997).

This gendered role was based on cultural and social constructions and essentialist views of the 'good woman' (Miers 2000). In addition, the hierarchical structures of class, gender and ethnicity within nursing further shaped the gendered nature of caring within nursing and midwifery (Heagerty 1990). And while there may be some changes to the gendered role of nursing given the changes in female working lives and the entry of men into mainstream nursing (Miers 2000), gender continues to influence caring and expectations of nurses as women (Davies 2003). Gender is also present in the situatedness of clinical practice, that is, how gendered bodies are treated in clinical practice in everyday interactions. For example, Davies (2003) suggests that female doctors appear to find different patterns of interaction with female nurses to male doctors and, in particular, facilitate less dominant and deferent doctor–nurse relationships. The history of nursing suggests how gendered nursing roles may influence women's preferences for female nurses as chaperones by socialising women into expecting cultural gender roles in patient–nurse and patient–doctor relationships.

However, in this chapter, I argue that these explorations of gender only take us so far in our understanding of the role of the female chaperone and what it may reveal about our understandings of nursing. I argue that the concept of embodiment may be more useful in understanding the effect of a gendered role such as a female nurse as chaperone in clinical practice.

Managing intimacy and emotions

Activity:

Many of you will have experience of chaperoning which may not be entirely positive. Make a list of these negative experiences and then see whether you can make a comparable list of the positive aspects of chaperoning.

Think of a patient where chaperoning was important and note down what aspects of chaperoning were difficult to provide.

Embodiment

Embodiment

Merleau-Ponty (1962) argued that the body is more than the physical object and suggested the concept of embodiment to understand the integration of the mind and body (Ettore 1998). In his theory of embodiment, consciousness can only be understood through the lived experience of the body or perception. The body is neither objective nor subjective because it is continually, mutually shaped or constructed through perception in each particular social and cultural context. Perceptions are reflective thoughts or judgements, which bestow meaning upon the world and are grounded in experience. Csordas (1994) emphasises that neither the mind nor the body is pre-eminent in a phenomenological understanding of the body. Rather the body is a biological, material entity and embodiment is the perceptual experience of engagement of the body in the world. Even this phenomenological body may be reduced to the status of an object under the gaze of another such as when an invasive technique is performed by a doctor, because the observer does not see the body as a person or experience it as a subject (Espeland 1984). In some situations, the gaze of another or the invasion of a private bodily space can be mitigated by the reason for being observed or subjected to a technique as when a doctor treats our body with our consent (Espeland 1984). Or, as Crossley (1996) suggests, embodiment may be thought of as our experience at two levels by way of our sentience (experiencing the body subjectively) and sensibility (being the object of an experience).

The public/private body

These analyses of the body allow us to explore ways in which the body and embodiment are socially, culturally and historically constructed (Csordas 1994). They also allow us to begin to integrate the body and embodiment into health care practice. As well as these mainstream approaches, feminist theories are informed by phenomenological approaches to the body (Young 1984; Grosz 1994) and others have recognised the absence of the female body in male theories of the body (Schildrick 1997)[13.] At the same time, other feminists have developed theories of political and social control that is exerted over the gendered body through medicalisation (Haraway 1992; Rose 1993; Schilling 2003). I have used a feminist phenomenological approach to understanding the body in this chapter. Ettore's (1998) work is an example of the approach I am arguing for, which integrates the body and embodiment in clinical practice. She argues that the processes and discourse of medicalisation have made bodies visible as empirical objects. This process of objectification is possible through medical technologies such as X-rays, blood tests and ultrasonography, which are the primary focus of medical investigations and treatments in ARTs. These technologies make bodies visible and have allowed medicine to understand them as empirical entities. This has meant that female bodies have become increasingly objectified and valued as gendered and reproductive bodies through medical technologies (Schildrick 1997; Meerabeau 1999). By this I mean the female body has become increasingly objectified as a reproductive body in ARTs rather than, potentially a body that cannot be or chooses not to be reproductive or capable of reproduction.

A further development of these analyses of the body and ARTs has focused on how medicalisation alters private and public spaces within the body (Price and Schildrick 1999). For example, Synott (1993) argues that the body carries a wide range of meanings and is polarised morally between male/female, old/young, beautiful/ugly, fat/thin, black/white according to cultural values. It is also internally polarised between private parts like the genitals and public parts like the face. Franklin (1997) argues that in in vitro fertilisation, an ART practiced on the body,

[13] Phenomenological approaches developed from a philosophical method of inquiry developed by Edmund Husserl, which investigates consciousness or the lived experience. Other writers in this tradition include Alfred Schutz and Martin Heidegger.

reproduction becomes possible with the help and assistance (intervention) of others. Therefore, private becomes semipublic or, at least, exposed to the gaze of a professional who is not in an intimate, social relationship with the woman (or man).

In this chapter, I start with the view that ARTs offer men and women the possibility of attaining biological parenthood while I recognise the potentially damaging effects such medical processes may have. Increasingly, more recent feminist writers argue that women's experiences of embodiment are not fixed and that there are changing spaces of embodiment for women during the states of pregnancy, infertility, ARTs and menopause (Grosz 1994). Ettore (1998) argues that the boundaries between bodies and society are changing and that this re-boundarying may be forms of restructuring power relations between the doctor and the 'ill' person through an acknowledgement of the embodied experience. This chapter adds to this view of the changing nature of women's embodiment by exploring the experiences of embodiment for infertile women seeking ARTs and the impact of the role of the female nurse as chaperone on our understandings of, and meanings attached to nursing in the gendered field of fertility nursing. I argue that acknowledging women's preferences for a female nurse as chaperone might be a way of coping with intimate, invasive medical procedures through the acknowledgement of an embodied experience which is mutually and unconsciously constituted as subjective and objective.

Activity:

Make a note of how you would describe embodiment after reading to here.

Try to explain the concept of embodiment to a colleague to see whether they find it useful to understand issues which arise in nursing practice.

Embodiment and infertility

Embodiment and infertility

I shall now discuss my interpretation of women's experiences of their lived bodies during investigations and treatments for infertility. I suggest that women describe their bodies during ARTs as healthy: abnormal, temporal and failing.

Healthy: abnormal bodies

Irrespective of diagnosis, many of the women said they felt healthy, looked healthy but felt abnormal, as they did not have children like their contemporaries. Wallach (1980:405) has described these feelings as 'being normal yet infertile'. As Dawn explained, her general practitioner had refused to accept that she was unwell as she looked healthy. It was 'only that I didn't fall pregnant' that she was referred to the clinic. This embodied experience of the differences between the external appearance of the body (sensibility) and the internal sensation of their infertile bodies (sentience) was a feature of infertile women's experiences:

> But you know you're dealing with people who are ill or frightened or whatever and they're not their normal selves. ... And something like this you're not ill [emphasis] but at the same time it can be, it can go on for so long and it's frustrating because there's a limit to what can be done. A lot of it's to do with the time of the month and so on. You're not sure if it's going to work. [Quietly.]

> So I've known that I will always have a problem. So it's not come as big a shock as someone who's probably been healthy and wonderful for all of their lives and then suddenly this happens to them.

> It's not like you're ill. You come in as a well person. And you're having a treatment that doesn't really make you sick. You're just a normal person. They're treating something which should happen naturally

Temporal bodies

For many patients, infertility changed their experiences of their bodies temporally and increased their experience of sentience and sensibility of a female body by sensitising them to their menstrual cycles. These were experienced subjectively as painful or disappointing (among other descriptors) and objectively as a recorded fact. Every month, time was spent waiting for a menstrual period, waiting for investigations and treatments to be done:

> Don't know how long it's going to take. And now I've been up here, it's been 3 months since I've been coming this time. I'm

still not pregnant. So you think it's 3 months, it's not wasted.
In 3 months, time just flies. Months come around and go.

They wanted to start treatments to 'speed things up' but after each investigation or treatment cycle were forced to wait for results and described this as 'just waiting'. Time was not within patients' control but experienced as subject to their bodies' internal working. This is graphically expressed by one woman, who on leaving after an intrauterine insemination (IUI), was asked if she wanted to book her next cycle. She said,

Oh that's no problem. It [her period] comes as regularly as clockwork.

The end of a cycle could spell the end of hope and the beginning of another round of waiting and hoping. Karen, Nita, Rebecca, Tracey, Ruth and Dawn, who had undergone failed treatment cycles, described time taken between cycles being a way to come to terms with failure. Failure was tolerated because these women had hope in future cycles, which were booked as part of their treatment protocols:

And just because my follicles were 22 mm I felt like you know 'Oh great'. Its really nice and important because if you've had months where nothing's happened and it's so she's very encouraging rather then otherwise. And this is nice because this is on the National Health because you know if it doesn't work this time then that there'll be a next time. They just say 'Oh well, we'll do this next time'.

The time spent attending the clinic and having treatment was not isolated time or time which could be forgotten. This time spent waiting for a pregnancy also became part of a baby should the treatment be successful and the absence of a baby, which became embedded in patients' lives as Dawn describes:

Because you've waited so long and infertility's a part of you and the baby's history. You never forget the infertility.

Failing bodies

Age was a powerful reminder for women of getting older, of declining fertility and of wanting children before they became too old to appreciate them. Four of the women explained their worries about ageing and failing bodies:

My lowest moment was when the private treatment failed and I wasn't on the NHS and I went to a party and every woman there was either pregnant or had children and they were all my age group!

It [residence] determines so much whether you're going to get NHS treatment and what age you're going to be allowed to have it until. You know I've friends who are 35 now and can't get treatment because of where they're living.

I know you can have children after 35 and everything but it would be nice if you could fall into the age they say is the best.

And I am worried about my husband's age as well. He's older now and you've got to think of him. You don't really want to leave it until he's much older.

These infertile women's experiences of time and their ageing bodies seemed to imply a heightened awareness of a changing, lived body but in their case, a failing, lived body whose purpose was increasingly uncertain as treatments failed (see also S. Williams' (1997) discussion of the uncertain body). Patients' concern with time and treatment cycles seemed to be an embodied experience of sentience and sensibility as they waited for each monthly, bodily change and each new or repeated medical intervention to relieve their uncertainty over their future. Their experiences of their lived bodies seemed to be constructed through technologies as described by Shildrick (1997). But in addition, their embodied experience included an absence, the baby.

I have described infertile women's experiences of embodiment during medical procedures in the AR clinics. I will now develop my analysis of the data in a discussion of the effects of such experiences on women's views on the role of the female nurse as chaperone and then consider how this extends our understanding about nursing.

Women's preferences for a female nurse as chaperone

Women's preferences

I have already discussed in Chapter 2 how patients viewed being a woman as a positive attribute of nurses because they believed that female nurses were better placed to care for and empathise with their experiences of infertility. Indeed, this is a striking feature of both data sets that being a woman was important for the nurses as well as the patients.

Another significant aspect of the data from study 1 is how the intimate nature of the task shaped the experience of the body for infertile women. Intimacy in the nurse–patient relationship has been extensively written about in the nursing literature (Menzies 1970; Savage 1995; Allan 2001, 2002). The investigation and treatment cycle for infertile women seeking ARTs is highly intimate and intrusive not only because it deals with intimate areas of the body for both men and women (Allan 2005, 2007a). It also deals with an intimate ontological area of being a man or woman who is unable to conceive and bear children (Pines 1993; Raphael-Leff 1991; Christie 1998). The following quote suggests just how intimate and invasive the investigations and procedures could be and the pressure women can feel placed under in the clinic:

HA: *Have you been examined internally?*
Pt: *Yes.*
HA: *And has that been done by a woman?*
Pt: *Well, it was my choice to be examined by a woman because I have the problem. I didn't want to let a man near me. When I had this operation at the EGA there was one student there, and the doctor asked me if I didn't mind having him in while I was having my operation, and I understood that he had to learn but it was only one student so I said okay.*
HA: *But you would prefer a woman to examine you?*
Pt: *At this point. I did think this a few moments ago and when I met Dr x and he wanted to examine me but I didn't want him to. But he was very good and I felt safe.*

When describing the sensations and thoughts they experienced during medical procedures, women stated preferences for female nurses to chaperone them during intimate medical procedures. Women's preferences for a female nurse as chaperone have not been addressed in the literature in the context of ARTs. An expressed preference for female nurses by women in this study was evident as the following quotes illustrate:

If there was a male nurse, they'd be doing their best. ... I think they'd probably have more understanding because they're female and I think I could discuss things better purely because they're female.

Managing emotions and the body in fertility nursing

It's all about the caring role and I'm sure a man could do it as well but ... you can accept a male doctor but not a male nurse. We are different [men and women].

They've been doing it for an awful long time ... so they've seen an awful lot.

Do they generally choose more experienced women and older nurses maybe for the delicate nature of this field?

These quotes suggest that women wanted female nurses to chaperone them during intimate examinations by doctors and that, generally, they wanted older women who have had some life experience and may have had children themselves. The question remains whether women wanted a female nurse as chaperone or an untrained female attendant such as a healthcare assistant. While the argument can be made that chaperoning requires skilled observation and a knowledge base and may lead to skilled interventions (Whittaker 1993; Allan 1999) [see also Chapter 4], the women were not clear about the difference between health care assistants and nurses and whether there were health care assistants working in the clinic. The majority were unaware and had not been informed of the difference between a trained nurse and an untrained health care assistant. They therefore only referred to nurses.

The women were, however, quite clear about the differences they perceived between doctors and nurses. Women differentiated between the doctor's role in the clinic and the nurse's. Their roles were perceived as having different foci: the doctor's being to diagnose and to treat, the nurse's being to work with the doctor, to care and be there to support patients. Women saw nurses as closer to patients in the sense that nurses understood what patients were experiencing and could communicate with them because of their personal qualities, their gender, the types of activities they carried out for patients as they arrived and the intimacy of their relationships with nurses. Women identified caring with nurses rather than with doctors and believed that nurses understood their experiences as women:

You must have a predisposition to want to relate to people anyway if you become a nurse. I don't believe the same is true of doctors because I think some people forget that it's a scientific discipline but that there are human beings with emotions that they are dealing with. But certainly with nursing, I'd find it very strange if they weren't interested in you as a person.

I suggest that the role of the female nurse as chaperone and its acceptability for female patients is shaped by expectations of gender, nursing and caring, which both challenge and reinforce notions of gendered caring and the gendered role of nursing. The role of female nurse as chaperone is therefore based on a perceived, shared gendered subjectivity that challenges the dominant patriarchal model of professional development inherent in nursing (Davies 1995). It is also potentially transgressive because it challenges the skills agenda and the mind–body split upon which skills training is based.

Discussion

The data presented in this chapter suggests that women experience embodiment of the infertile body both at a subjective and at an objective level. That is, they experience the body as an object acted upon through medical techniques and processes and as a body split into parts such as gametes (the eggs), postcoital fluids and hormones. They also experience the body as a subjective, lived body during the medical procedures in the unit, during the menstrual cycle and outside the clinic when interacting with fertile women (as suggested in Chapter 6).

However, the data in this study suggests that the objectification of the infertile woman's body might be less traumatic and oppressive than the feminist literature on the body argues (Schildrick 1997). Women consented to the procedures they were offered; the women and staff mutually managed a difficult social situation, that is, sexually invasive medical procedures, through the acceptance of the medical model as a way of understanding both infertility and the potential conception of a baby.

Medicalisation was accepted by both women and staff as the proper and expected way to proceed in the clinic. While there was discomfort in objectifying the body and performing intimate bodily procedures, women coped with these situations by assigning a shared gendered subjectivity to the female nurses. I argue that women made assumptions about nurses based on gendered notions of nursing and caring, which led to a shared subjectivity based on their identities as women and that this shared subjectivity mediated the objectification of the medical procedures and the medicalisation of their bodies. However, this gendered subjectivity was not expressed to female staff, and staff as well found emotions difficult to express and manage in the clinics (Allan 2001, 2002). Likewise, staff did not minimise women's discomfort through sharing gendered experiences but through their participation and roles in medical procedures (Allan 2001, 2002). As Menzies (1970) argues, it is at this level of unconscious work that nurses effectively care for patients and it is in more recent psychotherapeutic work that these unconscious processes used in caring are being recognised (Fabricius 1995; Savage 2003).

The role of the female chaperone may be understood as a response to the management of the medicalised body which women found 'unpleasant' and 'not nice'. The role is largely unacknowledged and hidden and, I have argued, is based on an implicit shared gendered subjectivity between female chaperones and female patients. While the role has recently been acknowledged (RCOG 1997), it is discussed within a framework of surveillance. The role of the female chaperone is seen as offering a third person, who is potentially able to 'protect' the patient from an implied sexual threat (Croft 1999). This analysis is superficially attractive because it assumes that the presence of the chaperone offers protection for the doctor in a medico-legal sense. However, it fails to explore the extent to which the female chaperone's presence increases the potential for self-regulation or governmentality to establish and confirm professional boundaries and ordinary sexual etiquette (Foucault 1979). And once again, this analysis reduces sexuality to the heteronormative model which ignores both the complexities of gender and sexuality for both men and women and the potential for acknowledging a shared gendered subjectivity in nursing practice.

It is true that the women did not express these preferences very often to doctors or nurses and this suggests several interpretations. It could be that the medicalisation of the clinic was oppressive and that there was little scope for expressing such a preference. However, clearly some women did do this and were accommodated. In one of the examples above, a male doctor was able to overcome a woman's anxieties around gender by acknowledging the woman's concerns and asking a female nurse to accompany the woman during his examination. It could be that these preferences were insufficiently strong for the women to express them.

However, there were examples where, again, women felt that the medical procedure was not handled sensitively and wondered if a woman could have handled it better. It could also be that these preferences were not expressed unless they were felt to be unmanageable. That is, if the clinical context and the discomfort this caused became intolerable then women might prefer a female doctor, but were able to tolerate a male doctor accompanied by a female nurse.

Implications for the role of chaperone

The implications of this data around women's preferences for female nurses to accompany them during such procedures are that increasingly NHS staff are under pressure to manage resources, and there is a risk that the traditional role of a chaperone during such procedures might be restricted or eliminated. As one nurse suggested, she felt under pressure from her nursing manager and the female consultants to stop chaperoning but she felt it was necessary and appreciated by patients:

> That way you get the confidence of the patient and they get to know you and if you try to help them to relax and relieve their pain, they sort of get to know you. And next time it's easier for them especially if they get the same chaperone.

However, while a female doctor or nurse might have lessened the discomfort in sexual terms for a patient, she did not necessarily remove the sexual nature of the examination or the associated discomfort altogether as Whittaker (1993) also argues. By denying that patients need chaperoning or a nurse accompanying them during a procedure performed by a female doctor, female doctors and their patients may be deprived of the support and comfort that this nurse refers to and that patients expected during an intimate examination.

Seeing a sexual threat arising only between heterosexual professional–patient interactions is common in medicine and nursing (Lawler 1990) and needs further exploration (Miers 2000). The question also arises as to why a female health care assistant cannot act as a chaperone. I argue that the skills and knowledge base underpinning nurses' actions and activities, such as observation, are required for this role (and discuss this role in more depth in Chapter 4). More recently, I have argued that even where a nurse undertakes a 'medical' task such as embryo transfer (Allan & Barber 2004), the nurse chooses to have another nurse chaperone the patient to provide this level of skilled observation and support for both the nurse performing the task and the patient, rather than a health care assistant.

In situations where nurses are taking on advanced roles in ARTs (Barber *et al.* 1996), the caring role associated with female nurses may be delegated to untrained staff or omitted altogether (Allan 1999). This implies that female embodiment itself is insufficient to justify the female chaperone role. And the data suggest that it is the gendered role of nursing as well as gendered caring that is identified by women as key to their needs during medical procedures. In some clinical situations (Allan & Barber 2004), the nurse undertaking an extended role is accompanied by a nurse who performs a traditional, caring role, which suggests that it is female embodiment as a nurse which is key to women's concerns. The potentially transgressive nature of the female nurse as chaperone is because the nurse acting as chaperone focuses on traditional female nurturing skills along with the observation skills I have described. This way of being a nurse challenges the skills agenda because it locates the nurse's expertise in her shared subjectivity as a woman and her ability to provide 'basic' nursing skills rather than technical expertise which underpins advanced nursing roles. This shared subjectivity is also trangressive because it uses an embodied approach to integrate mind and body in nursing practice through focusing on shared bodily experiences and subjectivity.

Conclusions

The role of the female chaperone is clearly ignored in the literature and I argue that this is because it appears to reinforce notions of gendered caring associated with traditional nursing. As Davies (1995) has argued, nursing is placed in a predicament because of its gendered position within health care.

This data suggests that women express a need for a traditional female nurturing or caring role during intimate sexual examinations. This sits uncomfortably with nursing as a gender-sensitive profession, which increasingly asserts its identity as a skilled, knowledge-rich profession within modern health care (Miers 2000). Additionally, in ignoring women's experiences of embodiment and focusing on the body as an empirical object, nursing continues to deny the emotional content of the clinical encounter and the need for recognition of this for the patient and their need to be cared for and contained (Fabricius 1991a, 1995). In developing nursing roles and reducing the time spent in traditional chaperoning duties, nursing has delegated skills which are valued by patients to health care assistants and further reduced the opportunities for providing supportive, emotional care. As I argued in Chapter 4, hovering and being there, along with chaperoning, offer the potential for the nurse to respond to patient need. If the nurse is no longer with the patient, she cannot observe, assess and respond. By ignoring women's preferences for female chaperoning, nurses avoid the arguments around gendered caring that are uncomfortable, to follow a model of professional development based on the male dominated professions of medicine and law.

The implications of this data suggest that there is room for further studies into the effects of gender on interpersonal aspects of health care delivery, as Hartigan (2001) argues. This data challenges notions of patriarchal professionalism prevalent in nursing which seek to move away from the traditional, gendered role of the nurse. The data also suggests that an exploration of the effects of gendered caring in advanced nursing roles would be illuminating in understanding how changing nursing roles and contexts of care affect women's care. This is the focus of Chapter 8 on advanced roles.

Reflection:

Have patients ever discussed their feelings and responses to infertility with you?

What reactions have you experienced after reading this data?

How far is it possible for women to choose the gender of their nurse?

Do you agree that they should be able to do this?

Do female nurses bring something to the woman–nurse relationship that men cannot?

Is sexual threat during an intimate examination a difficult area for you to address in your practice with women?

Chapter 6
Experiences of infertility: liminality and the role of the AR clinics[14]

In Chapter 4, I described how, as a result of managing emotions in particular ways, the nurses' main role was to run the clinics; running the clinic involved being there to 'fix things up' and guide patients through busy clinics which were frequently chaotic and confusing. Patients described their reliance on nurses to guide them through their clinic visits and to direct them between departments during the same visit. In this chapter, I discuss the disorder and confusion which infertility caused these infertile women and the role of the clinic in tolerating the chaos infertility produced in their lives. Data from study 1 is drawn on to illustrate my argument that this chaos can be understood as arising from the experience of infertility as a period of transition when the transformation from a woman 'trying for a baby' to the pregnant woman has not happened naturally. I use an anthropological term liminality to describe this period of transition because it conjures up images of being on the threshold of something important which so many of these women felt themselves to be. I describe how the AR clinics tolerated these liminal experiences and provided spaces where chaos and liminality could be allowed.

I argue that the British experience I observed appears to diverge from the American one of self-help and support identified in the literature (Sandelowski 1995). The British women I interviewed did not draw on self-help or peer support to deal with infertility. The clinic therefore became a place where support could be offered as, increasingly, assistance with pregnancy for infertile people takes place in the AR clinics through assisted reproductive technologies (Franklin 1997; De Lacey 2002; Tjørnhøj-Thomsen 2005). The clinic offered some recognition of

[14] Adapted from Allan, H. T. (2007a) Liminality and the experience of infertility: the role of the clinic in creating a liminal space. *Nursing Enquiry* **14**(2): 132–139.

their experience. At the same time, the low rates of conception following assisted reproductive technologies meant that the clinic also reinforced the experiences of chaos and liminality of those women who remained infertile. I suggest that the AR clinics may provide a liminal space where periods of limbo and transformation can be tolerated, while at the same time a medical space that creates more ambiguity and uncertainty.

The findings discussed in this chapter show that infertility was described by women as a chaos or social dis-ease where infertile women's relationships with fertile women were experienced as emotionally risky. I suggest that the clinic established a relatively safe place for this chaotic state to be acknowledged and managed because it offered opportunities to make friends with other infertile women. Another way in which the clinic managed the liminal experience of infertility was through the biomedical explanations it sought for infertility and through its investigations and procedures. The clinic offered reassurances and hope for infertile women, which contrasts with their negative experiences elsewhere. It offered a liminal space to be infertile but at the same time, limited ways of working with infertility and coping with uncertainty.

Reflection:

Think of a couple who have had outside support, perhaps even support from a patient support group. In what ways was this support helpful in their experience of the AR clinic?

Would you feel comfortable informing a couple about outside patient support groups?

Infertility: a liminal experience

Infertility: a liminal experience

The concept of liminality was used by Van Gennep (1909/1960) to denote a ritual of transition between one social status and another — a *'rite de passage'*, for example between adolescence and adulthood. Liminality creates a space and time for this transition to take place (Czarniawska & Mazza 2003). It can be seen as a state of being 'in-between' (Warner & Gabe 2004) two distinct social identities. It is also a place of uncertainty and unease where the end point of an experience is not always known (Warner & Gabe 2004).

Van Gennep described three stages of a *rite de passage*: separation, transition and incorporation. Separation could describe the decision to 'try for a baby' when a woman seeks a medical diagnosis and potential fertility treatment in AR clinics; she separates herself from both the fertile and the non-medicalised worlds. Transition describes the period when she is under the care of the AR clinics and where there is no certainty as to whether she may become pregnant or fail to conceive. Incorporation describes the transition to a successfully confirmed pregnancy for some and the potential new identity as a pregnant woman and mother.

But, for the majority of women, incorporation describes the assumption of a new social identity as an infertile woman. In the final stage, if the woman becomes pregnant, the identity of the fertile, pregnant woman may be threatened by early miscarriage and also by lingering feelings of identity as an infertile woman (Sandelowski 1993).

For many states of liminality, such as in death and mourning rituals (Bloch & Parry 1982), this period of being 'in-between' is socially legitimate. So, when someone has recently lost a family member, time and space are given to them socially to recover – to grieve. However, the experience of infertility as a legitimate social experience is often denied by the fertile (Greer 2005; Miller 2005).

Sandelowski (1993) has described the experience of living with infertility as the 'color gray', an ambiguous colour which describes periods where infertile women are 'on hold'. Tjørnhøj-Thomsen (2005) has also used the concept of liminality to explore the experiences of infertile women. She argues that the state of 'becoming parents is a rite of passage which marks an important change in social status, relatedness and identity'. She argues that assisted reproductive technologies are sought by women to resolve the temporal disruption and disorder which affects their lives, and to break the 'liminal dimensions' of their lives. I argue in this chapter that medicalisation does not resolve these liminal dimensions; it enables the infertile woman to tolerate the ambiguity and uncertainty by providing hope while at the same time, it contributes to the creation of ambiguity and uncertainty. Becker argues that infertility is an illness and, like all illnesses, is a disruption in the normal pattern of life. She argues that 'disruption helps explain when things go wrong in people's lives, when events happen outside people's experience and expectations of their lives'. During this period of disruption, people live 'in limbo', searching for meaning and a way out of uncertainty. Liminal states are characterised by disorder, chaos and pollution, which ensue when the social order is turned upside down (Bloch & Parry 1982). The state of liminality manages the period when the social order is subject to change and volatility and is thought in many cultures to be a time of danger for people who are closely affected (Bloch & Parry 1982). Greil (1991) has compared the liminal states of death and funerary rites with the experiences of infertile couples. It is recognised that infertility produces uncertainty in relation to both diagnosis and treatment (Tubert 2004) and is socially stigmatised in many cultures (Greil 1991; Tjørnhøj-Thomsen 2005).

'Matter out of place'

One way in which social relationships and conditions are stigmatised is through appearing anomalous or as Douglas describes this phenomenon, matter out of place. Douglas (1966) argued that one reason periods of disruption and transition (like death and mourning) are chaotic and anomalous is that they pollute normal social relations; that is, they disrupt social relationships and make things seem out of place. One way in which ARTs place 'matter out of place' is the belief these technologies interfere with nature (Tjørnhøj-Thomsen 2005) and appear anomalous and out of place. The interventions used to diagnose and treat infertility induce moral repugnance (Chodorow 2003) and working with infertile women in AR clinics in the UK involves the practitioner in extraordinary tasks such as handling gametes, facilitating masturbation of the man, monitoring sexual intercourse and assisting conception. In many of these tasks, staff handle matter out of place. I argue that medical discourse and techniques have assumed a role that enables women to manage their liminal experiences.

Becker (1999) argues that infertility is a life event that disrupts the western emphasis on a linear unfolding of life and, as such, produces chaos. The ability to nurture others is an integral part of socialisation for American women 'because fertility is a basic and embodied expectation for most women, infertility assaults embodied knowledge and core sense of self'. Becker admits that this is an American cultural discourse that suggests that life is an ordered, continuous whole. Does it apply to the British context?

Infertility: a chaos in women's lives

The following quote from a woman in this study shows how infertility was experienced as a time when she questioned previously held understandings of the world – a liminal state where the world turned upside down. Infertility is described as a blow to her identity and her sense of life purpose:

> At the end of the day, if I'm not going to have a child, what are we here for?

Adela, a black African woman whose baby had died at a very young age and who had secondary infertility, expressed her sense of uncertainty and longing for an answer to her infertility, as well as her belief that her purpose in life had also been frustrated,

> I keep asking them 'what's causing these cysts?' But they can't, they don't tell me. It's like they're finding another thing. So that thing is making me more mad. There's nothing they can do, nothing. How can you go on with nothing coming out of you?

One of the ways infertility threatens these women's sense of life purpose is through the length of investigations and the uncertainty of the success. Some of the women in this study described infertility as being endless and uncertain:

> I can't see an end to it.

> You don't know what to expect.

> Will I get pregnant in the end?

To resolve this sense of uncertainty, women expressed a desire to have control over the infertility:

> I want to know what's going on!

Roberta expressed this most clearly when she said she expected a point in her clinic attendance when the doctor would say,

> 'Well, this is what we've found. This is what we can do for you'. And then I presume it's up to me to basically say 'Yes I want to proceed' or 'No I'm going to withdraw'.

Managing intimacy and emotions

Sandelowski (1995) has argued that infertility is a relative not an absolute and that infertile couples remain in a 'tenuous state of being' which is never fully resolved. Even when a live birth had been achieved, the infertility remains part of the woman's identity. Dawn, who had a son conceived with the help of superovulation, described this quite clearly:

> Because you've waited so long and infertility's a part of you and the baby's history. You never forget the infertility.

Disruption to relationships with other women

These experiences of disruption and chaos produced emotions that tested infertile women's ability to manage their relationships with fertile women and made them uncertain how to continue friendships and family relationships with fertile women,

> And if looks could kill, I'd have killed her. I don't want them [her friends] not to have them [babies] just because I can't. I'm happy for my friends to have them [mimics envy, changes her voice]. Just because they've got pregnant after 2 months of trying!

> Sometimes especially when I see the women who had their babies when I had my first child. They're all grown up kids now. It's really sad ... All my friends have children .... Even my sisters all have children ... It's really depressing. It's like you don't know how to do it [have a child].

> And when, say, this is the end of the road and you're never going to have children, what do you suddenly do? Start not visiting your nieces and nephews because they're babies or not seeing your friend because she's just given birth? It's part of life and you just have to accept that.

Four women found that relationships within the clinic could be helpful, in contrast to their relationships with fertile women. As Susan says when describing another infertile woman who she has met in the clinic,

> Everybody's up here for a reason and you can feel supported by each other ... [She's] been a great friend and we phone each other and talk.

Dawn described that her reaction to the difficulties of telling outsiders about her infertility was to:

Oh, talk about it to everyone and anyone who'll listen here.

An extract from my field notes reveals how these friendships emerged from the women's encounters in the clinic.

> Adela smiled at Dawn's baby while they were both waiting in the corridor. Adela asked Dawn 'Is that your baby?' Dawn was friendly. 'I know just what you're going through but you have to persevere. I'll see you next week if you're here.' She smiled again and Adela looked more relaxed. When I interviewed Adela, I found out that she found Dawn's baby reassuring because it meant she too had a chance of becoming pregnant.

I argue that these quotes show the impact of infertility for women's sense of self and life purpose and how difficult women's relationships with fertile women could be outside the clinic, even with friends and family. To avoid these 'outside' relationships some of the women participants relied on relationships within the clinic, which were built up informally to manage their feelings, and to give them hope of becoming pregnant and resolving the infertility. However, for others, such friendships were not started and infertility was managed privately,

> *I couldn't stand 'Oh what's happening?' and all that. That would do my head in ... people asking all the time. I don't want everyone to know my problem. I tend to go home and cry.*

Being infertile in the clinic

This private attitude was more common among the women interviewed: 11 out of 15 infertile women interviewed said they did not talk to other women and only one woman said she was a member of CHILD, the British self-support group for infertile people. This lack of membership of support groups was initially surprising given the work done in America on the use of self-support groups there (Sandelowski 1995). I explored this finding in interviews with Helen Field and Dr Smith, the clinic counsellors, who felt that patients did not on the whole disclose to other patients in the waiting room, participate in support groups or have a great awareness of support organisations, because they did not accept the identity of an infertile woman. This interpretation is borne out in the literature as one of the ways of managing infertility identified by Sandelowski (1995), Sandelowski, Holditch-Davis & Harris (1990) and Olshansky (1987) is to construct an identity as an infertile woman and choose whom to disclose that identity to (Matthews & Matthews 1986). Therefore, the counsellors argued that these women were reluctant to form support groups that would have labelled them as infertile and given them an explicit identity that they shared with other women.

However, another reason for the lack of membership of support groups could have been limited access and knowledge about such groups as the staff did not discuss support groups, national infertility networks or the Donor Conception Network (www.dcnetwork.org) during periods of observation, advertise them in the clinic, or have experience of any successful support groups. Indeed, the counsellors seemed to think that staff were antagonistic to support groups. Only one nurse said she thought support groups were valuable when questioned directly during an interview. The women might have been influenced by these attitudes.

Instead of peer support either in the clinic or in peer support groups, women generally managed their infertility privately and appeared stoical. The following quote sums up women's attitude to managing their infertility,

> Maybe if I was told there was no way I would have kids, it would affect me but it's a fact of life. You have to go [on] don't you?

Part of 'going on' was attending the clinic in the hope that an answer would be found to their infertility through medical interventions. Unlike Becker and Sandelowski's studies, the women in this study did not access self-help groups. The women did not refer to seeking help outside the clinic but only to managing the social consequences of their medical investigations and treatments and to making friends with other infertile women in the clinic. Nor did the staff refer to encouraging self-help or give examples of referring women to self-help groups for peer support. It may be that in this particular context, self-help was not compatible with seeking medical help. The role of the British AR clinics, in contrast to the American clinic, may therefore be more necessary in helping women tolerate ambiguity, chaos and liminality, as it offers a way of being in limbo.

Reflection:

Is chaos a useful way to think about the effects of infertility?

Do you witness chaotic feelings among your patients when they are infertile?

Medicalisation: tolerating liminality and creating ambiguity

Tjørnhøj-Thomsen (2005) argues that reproductive medicine attempts to create certainty where there is ambiguity. This arises because, as Becker (1999) argues, although infertility is not a disease, it is treated as one in biomedicine. She argues that biomedicine identifies physical 'defects' that cause infertility and these defects in otherwise normal, healthy people can accentuate people's sense of disruption and therefore liminality. Sandelowski argues that medicalisation and the primacy of curing remain unchallenged in infertility (1993). The primacy of cure ignores the fact that 'medical therapies for infertility rarely eradicate or even ameliorate any dysfunction' (Sandelowski 1993:243). Technological advances mean that the quest of infertile couples for a child now involves more options than ever before but not necessarily more chances of achieving the goal of parenthood. As Sandelowski (1993:248) argues, technology can be a boon and a burden for infertile couples as the possibilities of cure have increased but so have the risks: one of those risks is that 'technology may reinforce suffering' through uncertainty because decisions cannot be made. One explanation of the primacy of curing in infertility is given by Becker (1999) who argues that, when people's individual life circumstances do not fit cultural ideas about what constitutes normality, biomedicine can affirm women's convictions that becoming pregnant is what normal women do.

Medicalisation is the process by which biomedical discourses explain normalcy (Becker 1999) and cultural notions of infertility become bound up in scientific, rational explanations about illness. Despite the primacy of cure, which assumes a reason can be found and a treatment offered, 'treated couples typically remain

just as incapable of reproducing after therapy as before'
(Sandelowski 1993:243).

I argue that this situation, where women sought medicalisation
to both explain and cure their infertility, produced a tension for
staff that was managed through a set of conflicting beliefs and
behaviours in the clinic. These beliefs and behaviours were
accepted as the unresolved realities of practice; in other words,
practice was also a liminal state. Understanding and explaining
infertility within a medical framework were contradictory to staff's
private acknowledgement in their interviews and informal conversations during observation about the failure of medical fertility
treatments to provide higher success rates and even a diagnosis.
Much of the medical practice in the AR clinics, such as recording
menstrual calendars, sexual positioning, advice about food and
rest and intrauterine insemination were not based on sound
clinical evidence but were enacted for something to do in the face
of no evidence or resources available to treat effectively. These
activities were accompanied by comments by staff following
intrauterine and donor insemination such as, 'think positive
thoughts', 'cross your legs'. The following extract from my field
notes illustrates the ways in which staff managed the tension
between medical fact and subjective experience:

> A patient of Dr Graham's who presented with a history of
> missing one menstrual cycle and heaviness in her breasts
> attended for a routine appointment prior to further investiga-
> tions. She suggested she might be pregnant although she had
> not performed a pregnancy test. When this was done, and
> seen to be positive, Dr Graham suggested she attend in 2
> weeks' time when an ultrasound scan of her uterus would
> confirm pregnancy. The woman refused and said she
> 'wanted a scan that day because she wanted to know'.
> Despite Dr Graham arguing against this, the scan was
> booked for later that day. Dr Graham explained to me that
> having a scan at 'such an early stage was often counterpro-
> ductive but patients were impatient and wanted technologi-
> cal reassurance'. Therefore, she had felt under pressure to
> arrange one.

Dr Graham knew that performing a scan this early in the
'pregnancy' was not based on clinical evidence. She recognised

that such medical interventions and advice were irrational and unscientific but felt that she was pressured to order such procedures, as patients were unsatisfied if there were no interventions. Dr Graham explained that she felt pushed into such interventions because 'women wanted technological reassurance'. These practices reinforced infertile women's beliefs that medical technology could provide an explanation of infertility and control fertility.

Reassurance or uncertainty?

Technology also creates uncertainty, as the object of investigation, the human body, does not always give clear results. In the extract above, the woman sought an answer to explain the tentative physical signs of early pregnancy and therefore an end to uncertainty; she 'wanted to know' and have her pregnancy confirmed. However, Dr Graham knew that an ultrasound at this early stage did not guarantee that the pregnancy would survive and that a scan could be counterproductive.

Other staff also felt that technology promised certainty (as Dr Graham did) yet was unable to deliver this and therefore actually increased the uncertainty of the infertility experience. These fears of the creation of uncertainty through the use of technologies have been discussed in other areas of medicine (Porter 1990; S. Williams 1997).

Why were these practices performed? I suggest that staff used medical procedures to manage the potential of a confirmed infertility diagnosis and therefore the transition to the new social role of infertile woman. I suggest that the clinic managed the chaos of infertility through these comments and the use of technology because not to do so would be difficult emotionally for patients and staff.

Medicalisation also provided a way of understanding the key importance of the clinic as a liminal space in which roles were negotiated, discarded and accepted. Medical processes in the AR clinics managed the liminality and were imbued with social meanings, which were relevant to and shaped by wider social meanings around gender, sexuality, parenthood and procreation. Another example of accommodating conflicting professional/lay world-views occurred on another occasion during fieldwork:

Managing intimacy and emotions

> Suki took me into utility room and showed me a slide with sperms. She looked at them under the microscope and said: 'they look okay ... it only takes one you know'.

Suki expressed her hope that there would be a conception from the sperm recently inserted into the female patient. It was a common view expressed by staff that conception only takes one sperm and one egg. However, in the context of ACU (study site 1), where sperm and sperm function are analysed for quality and quantity and where egg quality and release may or may not provide a good quality egg for conception, it is understood biomedically that fertilisation is more complex than Suki's comment suggests. In this example, two world-views of fertilisation, the medical and the lay, are accommodated by Suki who was an experienced gynaecology nurse. Dr Graham did the same thing when she told patients to 'think pregnant thoughts' as she inserted sperm during an intrauterine insemination procedure. While this used to make patients smile and relax as they smiled, it also suggested other beliefs. 'Thinking pregnant thoughts' suggests that thinking positively is important to assisting conception, that there may be a psychogenic link in fertilisation. These conflicting world-views were accommodated by staff in their clinical practice in complex and contradictory ways.

The patients I interviewed were in the process of medicalisation; they sought a diagnosis and treatment rather than to remain childless or seek alternative therapies. As an observer and from patients' accounts, medicalisation was most obvious in staff's management of the 'body'. Patients were symbolically divided into bits of the body to be investigated, as their bodies were treated as objects, scrutinised to reach a diagnosis and treat the infertility (MacDonald 1993). The body appeared to be divided literally at cell level into gametes, separated from the person (depersonalised) and given over to professionals for scrutiny.

The consequence of accepting medical management in the clinic as a place that tolerated their liminality and where friendships with women were less risky, was that infertile women accepted liminality and a biomedical possibility of resolving it. I argue that they did this without realising that the clinic and biomedicine also shape their experiences and in fact, limit their choices for action. It restricts their possible choices because it offers only the biomedical model. Just how restrictive medical clinics may become is suggested in the recent consultation by the British government on the Human Fertilisation and Embryology Act. Point 27 (DH 2005, para. 4.40) 'invites views on whether the requirement on licensed centres to offer a suitable opportunity to receive counselling should remain a legal obligation'. The British Infertility Counselling Association has suggested that there is a danger such services will be withdrawn from the Act (2005). As Becker says, there is a tension between the effort to find a personally acceptable route out of disruption and restore order and the difficulties of doing this in the face of the moral force of normalising ideologies, one of which would be the medicalisation of infertility and the primacy of cure.

In addition, the uncertainty produced through the use of technology and biomedicine to resolve a complex social and medical condition such as infertility resulted in a set of conflicting beliefs and behaviours by which staff attempted to reconcile medical facts and subjective experience. This sense of uncertainty and conflict gave rise to a clinical practice, which was itself liminal and mirrored women's liminal experiences of infertility and medicalisation.

Conclusions

While the technological potential to investigate and diagnose infertility has increased, the treatment success rates have remained relatively low (Bennet & Templeton 1995). I link the ideas previously discussed in the literature by Sandelowski (1993), Becker (1999) and Forss et al. (2004) who argue that, rather than creating certainty, medicine creates a new meaning in the context of health and illness which generates ambiguity for patients. Medical procedures in infertility allow for the potential transformation from non-mother to mother, non-father to father, non-parenthood to parenthood, gametes to conceptus (foetus). Of course, they also fail, and men and women do not become parents (Sandelowski 1993). I argue in this paper that the AR clinics in the British context are used as a place for tolerating the disequilibrium created by infertility; a disequilibrium which threatens social cohesion and creates chaos in social relationships. The clinic manages the liminality through medicalisation and the use of technology, which in the end creates its own uncertainty and liminality.

Managing intimacy and emotions

Activity:

Drawing from your experience in clinical practice, note down the benefits of seeking infertility investigations and treatments. Now note down the drawbacks to seeking out medical help.

How does the AR clinic either help or hinder the potential resolution of infertility?

Does the AR clinic make the experience of infertility worse for women?

Part III

Contemporary advanced AR nursing

Chapter 7
Managing intimacy in fertility nursing [15]

In this chapter I discuss the management of intimacy and closeness in the nurse–patient relationship in fertility nursing which takes place within the outpatient rather than the inpatient setting. Until recently, fertility investigations and treatments have been initiated and undertaken by doctors with nurses' coordinating treatment cycles, providing patient information or education and supporting doctors as they perform medical interventions. There is a great variety in the roles nurses undertake from those who manage patients' protocols during intrauterine insemination (IUI) or donor insemination (DI) to those nurses working in an outpatient setting who would not describe themselves as fertility nurses per se. The data I presented in Chapter 4 showed how fertility nurses manage the nurse–patient relationship through being there in the clinic and hovering – activities which in essence are undervalued by nursing managers although I argued that being there and hovering are meaningful for both staff and patients. It is precisely the invisible work in such roles which is supportive for patients and indispensable for the running of the clinics.

In this chapter I focus on advanced fertility nursing roles where nurses undertake egg collection, sperm aspiration and embryo transfer. Debbie Barber and I chose to explore advanced nursing roles in fertility because these roles create continuous contact between nurses and patients that potentially offers opportunities for intimacy and closeness. The nurses we studied take responsibility for managing the infertile couples' investigations and treatment cycles with supervision from a medical consultant and an embryologist. They have a degree of autonomy to undertake

[15] Adapted from Allan, H.T. & Barber, D. (2005) Emotion boundary work in advanced fertility nursing roles *Nursing Ethics* **12**(4): 391–400.

what were previously seen to be medical tasks such as ovarian ultrasound scanning, egg collection and embryo transfer. The data suggest that such roles positively affect nurse–patient relationships in fertility nursing by increasing the level of continuity experienced by both nurses and patients. However, they do not affect previously observed ways of managing emotions or increase levels of closeness or intimacy.

From the data we argue that emotions in nurse–patient relationships are managed through a form of knowing the patient, which creates a feeling of closeness but at the same time maintains a distance or safe 'bounded' relationship with which both nurses and patients are comfortable.

Activity:

Draw up a list of your key tasks and roles in clinical practice. Mentally evaluate whether these allow you to develop intimate relationships with women and their partners. Make a list of both the things which facilitate developing intimate relationships with patients and those things which act as barriers.

The nature of emotional intimacy in nursing

Emotional intimacy

Menzies (1970) argued that nurse–patient relationships change 'ordinary' social relationships and that there is a need to manage the intimate and emotional nature of these clinical, 'non-social' relationships (Allan 2001, 2002). These emotions and the nature of the nurse–patient relationship may be different depending on the context of the clinical encounter such as the gynaecological examination (Meerabeau 1999) or the AR clinics.

Empirical studies have suggested that intimacy is constructed in nurse–patient relationships in different ways. So, for example, May (1991) observed nurses using superficial conversational exchanges as a way of becoming intimate; in study 1, I observed nurses often asking patients about their holidays, their social events and exchanging information about their social lives. Patients appreciated this informal chatting and saw it as a way of getting to know the nurses and settling into the clinic on arrival.

Managing intimacy in fertility nursing

Tutton (1991) argued that the nature of the task determines the level of intimacy; in other words, if a nurse assists a doctor performing a vaginal examination or performs one herself, she can use a variety of strategies to manage this intimate procedure. She can acknowledge the intimacy or choose to disregard it as a way of managing any embarrassment; she can use humour to dispel embarrassment or chat about everyday matters to avoid embarrassing silences.

Intimacy is defined in the literature as the opportunity provided in 'the basic work of nursing... for a psychological closeness or meaningful relationship between nurse and patient that may hold therapeutic potential' (Savage 1995:11). There are quite strong views as to what the nature of intimacy might be in nurse–patient relationships. De Raeve (2002) has written that there is a moral imperative for nurses to create trustworthy, honest and authentic relationships (this view comes from the ethic of care approach described in Chapter 2); for de Raeve, authenticity of feeling is the basis of nurse–patient relationships and can be judged by whether the speaker feels committed to what is being said and whether the recipient feels there is sincerity. She argues that the nurse–patient relationship is different to friendship but, nonetheless, remains trustworthy and authentic. De Raeve suggests that professional relationships that require professionals to modify or control their emotions are inauthentic and untrustworthy. Phillips (1983), however, has argued that authenticity and emotional closeness in professional relationships are unlikely given the nature of professional practice, which involves an emotional distance. 'Friendship is not a requirement of the relationship . . . [the professional] need not be involved with the [client]' (1983:37). Girard (1988) has also argued that there are limits to intimacy.

Therapeutic use of self

Both the theoretical and the empirical literature on intimacy are shaped by earlier debates over the nature of caring and the therapeutic use of self in the 'new' nursing as described in Chapter 2. There are many definitions of the therapeutic use of self in the nursing literature and much of this is normative, that is, it is overlaid with a moral view of what is right, acceptable or expected within society. From the discussion so far, it is a normative view within nursing that nurses care for and are close to patients even when contradictory evidence exists to show that nurses do not care and do not have close relationships with patients.

The discussion in this chapter of intimacy and self are based on nurses' awareness of and ability to experience and vocalise the relationship between patient and self. There appear to be boundaries between private and professional spheres and the therapeutic self, in this sense, is the relationship between the personal and the professional or public self. Professional socialisation in nursing has historically emphasised that emotions are private and should not intrude on a nurse's professional life. Nurses have learned coping mechanisms to hide their emotional involvement in patients' experiences and historically they have not been encouraged to empathise with patients or to experience and vocalise the relationship between patient and self. Recent writing on emotions and the therapeutic use of self in nursing have suggested that this self might now be encouraged in clinical nursing (see Chapter 2). These authors (Uys 1980; Forrest 1989; Mahlstedt 1991; Barber 1991) argue that feelings such as closeness, empathy, and unconditional positive regard are observed within the nurse–patient relationship along with actions described as supportive. In contrast, it has been observed that emotional closeness with patients is not universally practised. To understand these tensions and contradictory observations, Savage (1995) found that, while physical and emotional closeness and intimacy are values promoted by the 'new nursing', nurses do not necessarily facilitate relationships of 'emotional intensity' with their patients. Emotional distance is a characteristic of nurse–patient relationships that can be described as close but nevertheless have a varying degree of detachment. Savage (1995) interpreted Peplau's writings (1969) to propose a closeness that includes an emotional distance. This emotional distance is achieved through nurses working to construct a caring environment that is therapeutic for patients 'without great personal cost for the nurse' (Savage 1995:124).

Nurse–patient relationships have also been analysed using emotional labour (Smith 1992; James 1992). As discussed in Chapter 2, emotional labour is the 'management of feeling to create a publicly observable facial and bodily display; emotional labour is sold for a wage' (Hochschild 1983:7). In the fertility context, nurses' and doctors' work could be understood from an emotional labour perspective as face to face and front line contact with patients, where feelings are managed or transformed to finish the work of the clinic (as described in Chapter 4).

Hochschild (1983) argues that certain occupations use surface and deep acting to shape emotions in themselves and others. Deep acting is where an emotion is shaped to produce a genuine feeling in the worker and works by either exhorting a feeling or by making indirect use of a trained imagination. De Raeve (2002) questions whether deep acting can be applied to the nursing context because it questions the authenticity of emotions that she sees as the basis of moral nurse–patient relationships. We argue that nurse–patient relationships are not morally grounded in authentic emotions but neither are they fully explained through the theory of emotional labour. Instead, I suggested in Chapter 4 that emotional labour does not fully describe how emotions are managed in the nurse–patient relationship in fertility care. I argued that emotional closeness or distance may be best understood through psychoanalytical approaches to fertility. Following Menzies, Craib and Fabricius, I suggested that managing emotions in fertility work necessitates an emotional distance as a defence against anxiety around nurses' own emotions in response to patients' situations, that is, nurses' emotional response to infertility.

In the rest of this chapter I discuss how nurses managed emotional intimacy through drawing on the findings from study 2 which was an ethnographic study of advanced fertility nursing described in Chapter 1.

Activity:

Read: Menzies, I. E. P. (1970) The functioning of social systems as a defence against anxiety : a report on a study of the nursing service of a general hospital. London: Tavistock Institute of Human Relations.

Discuss this paper with someone at work and reach some agreement about Menzies' argument.

Managing emotional intimacy in fertility nursing:

The nurses working in advanced roles were responsible for coordinating a couple's journey through investigations and treatment as well as specific tasks such as egg collection, embryo transfer, ultrasound scanning as well as taking blood specimens and deciding on treatment protocols. They were supported through team meetings where protocols were planned and if necessary medical intervention was planned. So, in effect, in suitable cases, patients' care was managed by nurses acting with senior nursing and medical support.

The nurses in study 2 justified undertaking advanced nursing roles because they believed that they could improve patient care through increasing continuity of care by taking on medical tasks which had previously been performed by doctors (see Chapter 8 for further discussion of their reasons for undertaking advanced nursing roles). By integrating these new tasks into their coordinating role, there was less disruption of carer for patients, less disruption for the nurse in developing their relationship with the patient and therefore more continuous knowledge developed of the individual patient journey and experience. Being responsible and present during the whole patient journey meant that nurses got to know their patients which they saw as beneficial.

Developing relationships through the performance of medical tasks

In the following extract from the data, the nurse describes using her social skills based on an established relationship with the patient to set the patient at ease during a procedure:

> N: ... and you usually sort of get them to say hello at some point or if I know I can't see them, I say 'Well this is so and so she's going to be seeing you'. It's nice for them then to have seen that person and know that is who is going to be looking after them, but I think if you can follow your own person through then that is fab, and they do feel a little bit more relaxed um and even just sort of as far as putting a venflon in, they feel a little bit more relaxed because you've been there and done bloods on them before.
>
> ... and you can make a laugh about it then y'know because

you've that little bit of rapport so you can sort of say, 'God look at the state of these' and they'll be laughing and won't be sort of panicking about it, so they know you then and feel a little bit more relaxed.

R: *It's very important at that point isn't it?*

N: *Yeah, and then I think for embryo transfers and IUIs it's lovely for them to say, Oh are you doing it? Oh yeah, y'know – I'm glad you're doing it sort of thing, because although we probably say to them early on that we do everything for you whatever,*

R: *um,*

N: *I think they've blocked that bit out and just think 'Oh that's got to be a doctor obviously it's so difficult', but I think once they've had them done and know it's not difficult, it's like 'Oh was that it sort of thing?', and know you can do them.*

One way in which performing the medical task facilitated knowing the patient and continuity of care was simply that the nurse didn't 'leave them' as these nurses say:

R: *I think it's a unique position because um a lot of sonographers only see a patient once,*

N: *Yeah,*

R: *and they give them probably that bad news and they won't know what's gone before and what goes after*

N: *Which must be an awful job for them y'know not to know, it must be hard, a lot of the times they can't say anything to them can they?*

R: *no,*

N: *which I think is a good thing that yes we can, we're not leaving them,*

R: *what are the benefits of your expanded role?*

N: *You don't have to say, you're coming in on this day to have a transfer done but I don't do them so somebody else will do them. So they don't have to meet somebody different and I'm able to continue on and carry everything through now, when before I would just see them so far and now I'm seeing them on my own.*

Continuity of care was facilitated by undertaking advanced nursing roles and building on their knowledge of individual patients, which developed from performing intimate tasks such as egg collection, embryo transfer or ultrasound scanning. Performing the task at the start of an investigation package meant nurses had a chance to get to know the patient as this nurse says:

> N: *Most scans are done as part of an investigation package so I will ... with our investigation packages sometimes we don't necessarily have a consultation with the doctor at the beginning so I think it's again just a familiarity of maybe one of the first really invasive procedures that somebody's had done and it is somebody that they actually know,*
> R: *Yeah*
> N: *um and y'know that they will have usually met me already, they know you and I, I don't know it may be an assumption that I think in some ways again because it's an extended role but I am a nurse I'm quite happy giving that sort of care, perhaps a little bit more than treating it as a procedure to be done. It's a part of, it's one investigation of a number that I would be doing.*

And continuing to perform the tasks led to continued care and developing a relationship with the patient:

> N: *And it is useful when you then have those patients back to go through what the potential treatments are that you've actually been there and done and seen and, it enhances the sort of trust relationship between you and I think that something like a scan which may be somebody's first invasive technique they can be very nervous and worried ... absolutely, and y'know putting speculums in if it's somebody they know and trust and they're relaxed with, it's got to have a better outcome for them than being tense and nervous while having it done by maybe a doctor they've never met before. I think it is this trust and relaxation, I don't know whether that is because we're women or because we're nurses it's maybe a mixture of both ...*
> DB: *um*
> N: *um, but I certainly feel that it's the knowing and meeting somebody before you do something nasty to them.*

Using feelings

Nurses described responding to their own feelings as cues to the patient's experience. One nurse described being aware of her own feelings in the nurse–patient relationship while at the same time imagining herself in another person's shoes:

Managing intimacy in fertility nursing

The one thing that I always try to bear in mind if I'm giving bad news of any kind is, no matter how bad or uncomfortable it is for me, it's ten times worse for them.

Two nurses described using or being aware of their feelings to assess and manage difficult situations such as pregnancy loss:

You've a little bit of a hint anyway from what they're telling you. They'll have had some bleeding, a little discomfort and you tend to get an inkling and they themselves will know and they'll say 'Oh no, I don't think it's going to be there'.

You usually have a feeling if it's not going to be, so you prepare them for it beforehand and if it's not fine then they've had a bit of time to go through in their mind.

The nurses' descriptions of their relationships with patients were supported in the interviews with patients. Words and phrases such as 'forming a bond', 'feeling quite close', 'feeling comfortable with', 'being on the right wavelengths' were used by patients to describe their relationships with nurses. They said that these relationships developed from telephone support, the availability of contact with their individual nurse and the continuity with this nurse during treatment cycles. The descriptions of couples' relationships with nurses included:

She seemed to be genuinely really pleased. It was quite a personal thing.

We did very much feel they were on a par with us.

They treated me with respect.

Patients did not say that their relationships were different to other relationships they may have had with nurses, neither did they reflect on the new roles nurses undertook in the clinic. However, the nurses did comment on the effects of these new roles on intimacy and knowing. They believed that advanced roles increase nurses' ability to know and therefore to provide continuity of care for infertile couples:

I had one woman who, she didn't miscarry but she said she wished that I had been there. I wasn't the one who'd done the scan [to check for pregnancy]. She said, awful as it was and as awful as she felt, she wished it had been me doing the scan and telling her it didn't work.

You try to find someone [nurses] they click with and ... some [nurses] may not have started your patients but you pick them along the way or some patients end up being other people's [nurses] patients because that's who they feel confidence in. You can tell, just how willing they are to talk to you and how open they are about their daily life.

I certainly feel with patients I know I have a vested interest in collecting every single last egg they've got. It's very important to me; it's not a quick five minutes and I want to get out.

There was an awareness that managing patients through their cycles and co-ordinating their cycles also facilitated the relationship and made it different to doctors' relationships with patients:

N: *and attention, I'm not saying that doctors don't, but they don't usually all probably in a lot of set ups don't know the patients*
R: *no*
N: *they haven't lived through the preparation, had the ..., y'know they haven't had all that background history with the patient to make it as important to them*

The difference that continuity of carer made in the context of coordinating protocols and performing all the tasks within that protocol became apparent when describing a task like information giving:

Say you're doing an injection, you're not just doing that, you're asking them how they are and you're getting a bit of two way conversation going that enables you to pick up on any other problems which are there. So it's not just an injection, they've come for information, to build up a relationship with you. Whereas I think doctors see that as a task.

And I might spend their first visit only talking a little bit about IVF, I know I've got to get that information across at a different time, but I think it's trying to assess the level of information they need at that time which is the deciding factor, what each couple needs. There's no point if you've got a couple who are very nervous, who are not feeling familiar with medical terminology, it's a waste of time giving every little bit of information. It's a waste of time.

They don't want to be 'talked to' they want to be 'talked with' … I think that's what's important.

And what doctors don't do although Alan (the previous consultant) was very good. He would go in and say, 'Tell me why you're here' and that would be a good opening.

It wasn't what people expected. A lot of people expect to come for a consultation to be told what to do. And that's different in IVF because it's the couple's choice, it's not an illness that's going to kill them, they've got choices that only they can make. I think it's important that we get across … we help them tell us what those choices are and with some couples you can communicate information very rapidly to and with others you have to pitch it to their level and time.

Limits to relationships

Knowing patients in this continuing relationship was rather more complex than the data suggests. The nurses also believed that 'knowing a patient' contained a distance and was a professional knowing rather than an intimate form of knowing, as these quotes suggest.

We can never say we know the patient. We all get couples where the relationship has broken down and we knew nothing.

N: *I think this is probably going to sound quite dreadful, I think in some ways being, in some ways you have to be a little bit more detached doing surgical procedures, when you're doing sedation checks, I think you have to have an element of in some cases. It can be uncomfortable and you know that the procedure has got to be done, so you need a little bit of detachment. I think that comes or, it certainly came for me learning how to cope with pain during labour. I think to do your job properly you have to be, you have to also have some distance to know that it will come to an end but you've still got to, you can't be so involved that you can't do your job properly*
R: *um*
N: *Being detached is necessary. It's not detachment but saying I know it hurts but I've got to carry on.*

N: *Absolutely, I think a lot of the clients that come through, because you do see quite a lot of them sometimes, you do get quite friendly with them*

R: *do you find that makes it difficult in managing their care?*

N: *Um, not normally. I try not, I mean I know some nurses do occasionally see people out of work, but I don't feel that's appropriate for me*

R: *um*

N: *so although I'm very friendly with them at work, its still work and I leave it here*

R: *yeah*

N: *I think that's important.*

Distancing included recognising one's responsibility for one's own emotions. In the following quote, the nurse describes maintaining a distance by giving back responsibility for emotions to patients. She feels that the burden and effects of their emotions are sometimes too much to bear and suggests that infertile couples need to manage their emotions themselves.

They've got to accept responsibility for themselves, they're grown-ups at the end of the day. It's a big thing for them in their life and passing it back to them as well because it's hard for you then to accept all this responsibility for everybody.

This distancing was also a matter of respect for patients' rights to privacy:

Becoming too close to a person, they don't want that and I think you have to respect that.

While recognising these constraints on knowing and intimacy, a nurse describes her relationships and the degree of personal knowing that develops with patients as intimate to a degree determined by the nature of the clinical encounter:

It's not superficial because some of what they tell you is really intimate. I think you could describe it more like knowing a small core of that person.

Discussion

The data suggests that emotions are acknowledged and used in caring for patients and that using feelings is possible because of the continued relationship that is facilitated through advanced nursing roles which include performing previously medical tasks. Nurses' descriptions of their therapeutic use of self reveal one way of managing emotions, but they are also evidence of the presence of emotions in the clinic and the importance attached to them by nurses. In contrast to de Raeve (2002), we argued that the data does not suggest deep acting or that feelings or the management of feelings were inauthentic. Emotions are recognised and understood by these nurses to be authentic and the moral question for them is whether to take on responsibility for the advanced role that increases continuity of care within a 'bounded' relationship that facilitates comfortable levels of knowing and intimacy. De Raeve's emphasis on authenticity also does not capture other processes that could influence the management of emotions in nursing work. These processes may include Savage's idea of constructing a caring environment 'which is therapeutic for patients' (1995:124). They could also include utilising opportunities for intimacy within each clinical encounter; that is, opportunities for emotional closeness to patients are context bound as well as bounded by emotional distance and closeness. Our data suggest that nurses offer and that patients 'sense' something more than instrumental care, even when engaged in routine tasks.

One explanation for this situation could be that being able to perform medical procedures allows continuity of care for patients by nurses, and that the routine itself becomes meaningful because of the emotional relationship based on the continuous nurse–patient relationship developed during investigations and treatments. The performance of medical tasks facilitates a greater continuity of care and a shared sense of knowing and intimacy between nurses and patients.

None of the nurses described their relationships with patients as being emotionally close in terms of a display of emotions. Yet this did not mean that the nurses believed that their relationships with infertile patients were unlike other nurse–patient relationships and were dominated by medical tasks. They argued that their roles could improve continuity and support for patients and therefore increased how well they knew their patients and how intimate they were. They quite clearly justified their roles in terms of developing patient-centred care, which is in line with the current thinking. The critiques of new nursing roles have argued that the roles that involve medical tasks assume a hierarchy of knowledge, with medical knowledge being at the top of the hierarchy. Our data suggest that this is rejected by this group of nurses, who see their roles as developing from patient need rather than being imposed by management or from a desire to 'master' higher-status knowledge and tasks.

Boundaried relationships

One way of understanding the descriptions of their relationships with patients may be through a psychoanalytic understanding of the role of emotions in nursing practice. Nurses control their responses to maintain a position between emotional closeness and distance as a defense against the anxiety of the emotions, which they recognise as being present in the encounter with patients. This knowledge (consciously stated in the interviews) and the defenses (unconscious and not described) to which the nurses in this study appear to be alluding, may develop from the continuity of caring for a couple throughout their treatment cycles and result in what the patients call 'bonding'. Bonding or attachment arises from patients' need to form a dependent relationship with a significant other during a period requiring dependency such as infertility treatment. The nurses in this study appear to have managed both the dependency and the anxiety by conducting a relationship with patients that was neither too close nor too distant, but responsive to patients' needs while at the same time not damaging to the nurses themselves.

There is much that remains unknown in this 'bounded relationship'. For example, the extent of the personal and emotional work required to fulfil one's professional role and the knowledge that underpins this relationship is, we suggest, unconscious and unknown. It may be intuitive or nurses may be acknowledging their own feelings in response to the patients' own and responding appropriately to them. This, in itself, is highly skilled and developed through expert supervision. In this emotionally managed relationship, nurses may be able to distinguish their emotional responsibility from that of the patients, and forms of emotionally responsible practice may be identified in the future. At the very least, recognising the influence of the practice context on emotions and that responses are contextually and responsibly appropriate is essential. This may be the emotional response that de Raeve refers to when she speaks of authenticity (2002).

Managing intimacy in fertility nursing

One significant aspect of the data is how the intimate nature of the task shaped the nature of the nurse–patient relationship, and the forms of intimacy and knowing that were developed. The investigation and treatment cycle for infertile patients is highly intimate and intrusive because it deals with intimate areas of the body for both men and women, and with an intimate area of being a man or woman who is unable to conceive and bear children. The nurses recognised that, for some patients, the degree of intimacy in the physical sense shaped and restricted the level of intimacy in the social sense. The intimacy was focused quite specifically on a narrow area of the patients' lives and did not generally go beyond this. In this way, the task and the nature of the intimacy seemed to demand a nurse–patient relationship that was more distanced rather than intimate, as Girard (1988) argues. She suggests that medical and surgical patients require emotional privacy because their physical privacy is not maintained and patients cannot 'surrender both physically and emotionally' (1988: 28). Our data suggest that patients described closeness with nurses but not relationships that were emotionally intense; nurses not knowing that there were difficulties in couples' relationships could be an example of this. The nurse–patient relationship was based on social acquaintance rather than physical or emotional intimacy, although some degree of physical intimacy was required owing to the nature of assisted conception. This situation of enforced physical intimacy may have been why patients avoided emotional intimacy (as Savage found) and, indeed, some patients may actively reject an emotional intimacy by maintaining a distance from nurses in AR clinics. Some patients responded to closeness or intimacy when they judged it appropriate; for example, when they chose to come to the summer party with their babies.

Conclusion

We have argued that nurse–fertility patient relationships in advanced nursing roles where nurses take on technically advanced tasks (previously seen as medical tasks) are a vehicle for managed closeness rather than increased intimacy. We have argued that these relationships are based on an unconscious awareness of the potential emotions in the nurse–patient encounter; nurses offered and patients 'sensed' something more than instrumental care even when engaged in routine tasks. Our findings suggest that patients benefit from increased continuity of care facilitated by these advanced roles. In this case, continuity of care was provided by changes to nursing roles where nurses took on increased clinical responsibility for what were medical tasks. The advanced role increased continuity of care within a 'bounded' relationship that facilitated comfortable levels of knowing and intimacy. These nurses were able to effect this change by challenging received wisdom about the limits to nursing responsibilities and given orthodoxies about the nature of intimacy in nurse–patient relationships.

Reflection:

Having read this chapter, what conclusions do you draw about Menzies' original paper?

Do you feel the nurses in this study were correct in their descriptions of their relationships with women as having 'limits'?

Chapter 8
The nature of advanced fertility nursing roles: why do nurses undertake them?[16]

I have argued in this book that reasserting the value of caring in nursing practice through the role of chaperoning or hovering or being there for instance, might be seen as transgressive or challenging to some professional models of nursing practice as well as current health care policy because these roles appear to hark back to a former model of nursing (Carpenter 1993; Allan 2007b). These older types of nursing are understood to be merely supportive to doctors but actually they facilitate nurses to assist, support and respond to patients through being present. In this chapter, drawing again from data in study 2 which explored nurses' advanced roles in fertility nursing, I describe the ways in which nurses working in advanced fertility roles place the caring relationship at the heart of the role. I do this through exploring their reasons for undertaking advanced roles. On the one hand, these advanced roles require extra training as well as increased levels of responsibility and require the nurse to learn to perform tasks which are technically difficult. Of course, on the other hand, they offer the nurse increased levels of autonomy, control over her actions and continuity of care of specific patients. The findings from study 2 suggested that in undertaking such roles, nurses appear to need a moral narrative to justify their advanced roles. It is these moral narratives which form the basis of this chapter. I believe that these moral narratives are necessary for nurses because these roles appear transgressive in four ways:

1. They challenge accepted and expected ways of working with medical colleagues, i.e. as their support (as described in Chapter 4);

[16]Adapted from: Allan, H. T. & Barber, D. (2004) 'Nothing out of ordinary': Advanced fertility nursing practice *Human Fertility* **7**(4): 277–284.

2. They challenge current models of professional development because they reassert caring as part of an advanced nursing role;

3. They assert gendered caring, i.e. that being a woman in caring for an infertile woman going through ARTs is important for patients;

4. They challenge accepted theories of caring which assert that emotional closeness or intimacy is the goal of professional nursing practice.

Reflection:

Have you been asked to take on or train for an advanced role? Can you list the reasons why you were asked and why you considered or agreed to take it on?

Nursing workforce policy

Nursing workforce policy

The fertility nursing role currently includes a range of responsibilities from egg collection and embryo transfer to the outpatient nursing role of doctor's assistant (Corrigan 1996; Barber *et al.* 1996; Birch 2001; Hinks *et al.* 2002; Allan & Barber 2004; 2005). This variety of nursing activity is entirely in line with current nursing practice in the UK (RCN 2007; UKCC 1997; Daly & Carnwell 2003), that is, nurses' roles and responsibilities vary according to specialty, employer and professional development. This appears to me to be entirely congruent with the intentions of the Scope of Practice introduced in the 1990s (UKCC 1992).

It is claimed that the advanced role in fertility nursing can enhance continuity of care (Hinks *et al*, 2002), that nurses practice differently to doctors and are able to provide holistic care (Corrigan 1996; Birch 2001). Apart from a few papers (Barber *et al*, 1996; Birch 2001; Hinks *et al*, 2002), there is very little exploration of these issues in the fertility research literature. What is interesting in the debates within fertility nursing, and in other fields of nursing where similar roles are being developed (Williams 2001), is the claim by fertility nurses that they perform medical tasks in a holistic manner. They claim to be able to retain nursing's core values of caring and intimate care while performing what are technically skilled tasks (formerly medical tasks). This apparent contradiction between holism and specialism in nursing has also been noted in the role of nurse practitioners in primary care (Williams 2001). As I have argued in this book, this is a complex claim and was the stimulus for study 2.

These changes in nursing roles reflect wider debates at national and European levels over the future delivery of health care (Salvage & Heijnen 1997; UKCC 1999c; Bryant-Lukosius *et al.* 2004), in particular around workforce training and education, shifting care into the community and funding arrangements (DH 2008). There is concern both within the nursing profession and in government over the skills required for future health care delivery and, in particular, how different levels of nursing practice meet future health care needs (Manley 1997; Daly & Carnwell 2003; DH 2000; DH 2008). Advanced nursing roles (and other nursing role developments) are intended to make a valuable contribution to delivering effective health care and helping to modernise the NHS (DH 2000). However there is concern over the plethora of nursing roles being developed and the lack of agreement around the rationale for changes to nursing roles or even the titles by which new nursing roles are called (Manley 1997; Barber 1997; Daly & Carnwell 2003). There is also conflict and anxiety in the relationship between health care assistants and nurses over the delegation of practical, caring activities from nurses to untrained carers (Bradshaw 1995; Allan 2007b).

Changing professional boundaries

In the broader context of the doctor–nurse relationship and their respective relationships with patients, there is increasing tension between medicine and nursing around the changing role of nurses, particularly over the role of nurse practitioners (Salvage & Heijnen 1997; Ashburner *et al.* 1997; Williams 2001; Horrocks *et al.* 2002; Daly & Carnwell 2003). This tension exists despite the Government's encouragement for doctors to delegate some tasks previously defined as medical to nurses (DH 1997a) and in innovations such as NHS Direct (DH 1997b) and nurse prescribing (DH 2000). For example, *Agenda for Change: Modernising the NHS pay system* (1999); *Making a Difference: Strengthening the nursing, midwifery and health visiting contribution to health and healthcare* (1999); and *Working together: securing a quality workforce for the*

NHS (1999) and subsequent publications by the Department of Health (2008) all suggested that changes need to be made to how nurses' skills are used in future. It is proposed that nurses take on extended roles and medical tasks releasing doctors for higher level tasks (DH 1999; 2000; 2006; 2007). The professional bodies have endorsed these proposals (UKCC 1999b). Indeed, it was argued in *Healthcare Futures 2010* (UKCC 1999b) that the kind of problems which form the background of this study, concerning the nature of the caring role and the development of the nursing role, are going to deepen. However, as in Manley's work in intensive care and expert nursing (1997) and Williams' work with nurse practitioners in primary care (2001), careful attention needs to be given to how nursing roles are developed. As Manley says (1997) they need not be extended roles which are merely taking on medical tasks; they can be advanced roles which retain the core of nursing as Birch (2001) claims is the case in advanced fertility nursing roles. This position is not helped by the proliferation in nursing roles and titles (Daly & Carnwell 2003).

New nursing roles have led to changes in the doctor–nurse–patient relationship; historically the primary therapeutic relationship was understood to be that which occurs between the doctor and patient. In fertility nurses' descriptions of their advanced role in study 2, the central relationship is taken to be that between nurse and patient with the doctor remaining outside this relationship. In other fields of nursing, these changes have led to resentment by doctors at attempts of nursing to act independently outside this framework (Manley & Garbett 2000; Horrocks *et al.* 2002; Coombs & Ersser 2004). By acting outside the medical hegemonic framework, nurses are seen to challenge previously held notions of the therapeutic relationship between the doctor and patient. Boundaries between professional disciplines are therefore changed as nurses assert that the nurse–patient relationship can be as therapeutic as the medical relationship. Much of the research into the significance of continuity of carer has been done by midwives who have met resistance to their independence for many years. Although there is anecdotal evidence of this tension in fertility units, and some awareness from nurses that the changes in roles may threaten doctors, this is not explored in the literature (Barber 1996; Allan & Barber 2004).

The nature of advanced fertility nursing roles

Changes to nursing roles more widely have occurred at a time of media reports of patients' concerns that there is a lack of caring in the health services at the same time as a rapidly expanding range of technological and therapeutic interventions (Allan 2007b). Equally, there have been publicised reports of medical 'blunders' and an acknowledged lack of accountability to the public which have stimulated debate (see for example, Hugman 1998) as well as government action (DH 1999; DH 2000).

The Labour government since 1997 has sought to address these wider issues of labour shortage in several ways. It has proposed changes to nurses' career structure and pay scales (*Agenda for Change*, DH 1999; *Modernising Nursing Careers*, DH 2006; *Towards a Framework for Post-Registration Nursing Careers: A National Consultation*, DH 2008) to encourage nursing morale, recruitment and retention. It has encouraged nursing autonomy (Manley & Garbett 2000) through its recognition of the value of nurse-led initiatives in primary health care (Williams *et al.* 2000). Finally, its backing of 'consultant' nurses and its willingness to listen to nursing representation is widely thought to reflect government's political will to reduce the power of medicine and encourage a more accountable, consumer-orientated health service. Interestingly, nurses see themselves as being more in tune with patient demands for a more accountable and consumer orientated health service (DH 2000). The challenge for new nursing roles is to show direct patient benefit (Spilsbury & Meyer 2001; Horrocks *et al.* 2002) and resolve cultural factors such as barriers within multidisciplinary teams towards nurses leading decision-making (Coombs & Ersser 2004).

More specifically, the poor level of provision of fertility services in England and Wales (Souter 1997) and the historical evidence of the general lack of funding and access to infertility services (Hull 1992) add another dimension to discussions of labour shortages in reproductive health services. The shortages and related changes to nursing roles reflect questions over how provision of reproductive choices and preparation for parenthood are to be delivered and by whom. These debates have occurred at the same time as 'family' initiatives introduced by the World Health Organisation and the European Union (Doyal 1998) and reflect a wider awareness of reproductive health issues in policy terms. Lastly, these debates are in turn influenced by the concern over medical and nursing labour shortages, recruitment and training at European level (UKCC 1999c) and the restrictions to the free movement of workers between European countries (Salvage & Heijnen 1997).

There are three broad areas in the literature which provide the background to this study. The first is the United Kingdom Central Council's (UKCC) Higher Level of Practice Project (2002). This project analysed the different levels of practice and the new titles nurses have acquired following the publication of the UKCC's *Scope of Professional Practice* (1992), the *Future of Professional Regulation* (UKCC 1998) and the reduction in junior doctors' hours (DH 2003). The second area of the literature deals with the effect that role extension has on 'nursing' (RCN 2003). Role extension has not always been viewed as a positive development for nursing but as a delegation of unwanted medical tasks to nurses. The third area is the knock-on effect of higher levels of practice on the delegation of 'traditional nursing roles' to health care assistants (Davies 1995; RCN 2003). This delegation has raised concern over who provides nursing care as well as what care is provided (Warr 1998; Kitson 1999). The changes that these policy initiatives effected can be seen as an attempt to develop the future workforce of the health service (RCN 2003). Our study provides empirical data on the effects of these policies on fertility nursing practice and inter-professional relationships in one clinic in the UK as well as data on nurse–patient relationships in new nursing roles.

Activity:

What are the factors which drive forward advanced nursing roles?

What are the advantages for patients of such roles?

Can you identify any disadvantages?

The nature of the task

The nature
of the task

Our data suggests that changes to nurse-led practice may emerge when a belief exists among practitioners that the nature of the task demands changes to practice. This belief was expressed in the view that advanced nursing roles are a 'natural extension' of the nurse's traditional role,

> There's no way we are mini doctors. These are areas we are specialised in and we have more knowledge in these areas than a lot of doctors have and will have unless they work in the field full time (N1)[17]

To justify changes in nursing roles, N2 describes her belief that caring for infertile patients can be improved if the same nurse cares for a patient by performing medical tasks during a treatment cycle,

> It's ... a familiarity of one of the first really invasive procedures that somebody's had done. And it is somebody that they actually know ... it's an extended role but I'm quite happy giving that sort of care, perhaps a little bit more than treating it as a procedure to be done. It's a part of, it's one investigation of a number that I would be doing [for that patient]. (N2)

This quote indicates that N2 believes that being a nurse means that she approaches tasks differently to a doctor. The medical consultant also believed that experienced, specialist nurses brought something qualitatively different to the task.

> You can see the advantages of somebody known to the patient, who's probably scanned the patient on several occasions, and having them be responsible for the egg pickup. The perceived benefits to the patients seemed to be continuity of care, relaxation and predictability [of the nurse attending them] that came from the nurses doing the procedure. Since they were technically competent, it seemed an obvious and natural development ... (Consultant 1)

Another reason Consultant 1 gave for specialist nurses being safe to take on advanced roles was that their role was the key focus in their professional lives unlike a registrar gaining experience of

[17]N1, N2 etc. refer to nurse participants.

fertility en route to his or her consultant's post.

> *They're much better than junior doctors because they stay longer and become more skilled and they regard it the pinnacle of their clinical practice. Whereas [it] simply being some boring stage on the road to something more exciting.*

While the data suggest that the role changes were viewed as a natural and unforced area of development, nevertheless, the nurses described the process of transition between roles too. Woods (2000) argues that expectations and meanings attached to such transitions are influential in shaping role transition. The data in this study suggests that the positive expectations of the medical consultant and the negative expectations of the wider fertility world were influential in shaping how and when such transitions were introduced. For example, N1's decision to delay egg pickup until NHS clinics had started doing the same:

> *It was knowing someone else had done it first and had got approval within an NHS Trust. That gave us the confidence that we would be able to get through the loopholes to actually get on …*

But even when such transitions were acceptable and expected, some nurses did not make the transition for personal reasons.

> *I think it's important that people aren't forced into doing things that y'know, take on skills they're not entirely happy with.* (N4)

Woods (2000) further argues that certain types of role transitions are qualitatively different to others. He suggests that, rather than simply extending roles as nurse practitioners do, where the nurse learns and adds new skills to her repertoire, the advanced practitioner needs to deconstruct and reconstruct her role. This deconstruction and reconstruction involves re-framing her attitudes, behaviours, identity and relationships in the new role. Our data suggests that, as this deconstruction and reconstruction happens, nurses formed their narratives to justify these changes. These narratives are reflections on how the role change has affected their understanding of being a nurse, their knowledge base and their ethical explanation for their new roles and responsibilities in their relationships with patients. As well as a belief that their new roles were justified and qualitatively different to medical roles, three factors were identified as having influenced these role changes:

- personal factors
- interpersonal factors
- socio-cultural factors.

Personal factors

The data suggest that personal factors such as the individual nurse's emotional preparation for fertility work were central to nurses' explanations for their new roles. The nurses felt that their experiences of being women caring for women enhanced care. N2 described her experience,

> *Um, I think just generally having experience of being female, although I haven't got children, you know the delight and joy that babies bring to a lot of people and therefore being at the other end of things people who can't have children, from my point of view a field that would be very difficult to come in as a young inexperienced nurse. I think a new qualified nurse would find it quite difficult.*

Personal factors also included honesty and responsibility. If the nurse took on new roles such as scanning, she also had the responsibility to be honest with patients,

> N2: *I think there isn't any one approach to telling somebody bad news.*
> Interviewer: *Um.*
> N2: *Um, other than being, trying to be sympathetic but people may not want you there at that immediate point. I think to give them the news it's sometimes easy when you've got a relationship with somebody to think, Well yes I know y'know, give them the news. Leave them alone for a few minutes with their partner and then come back.*

In the following quote, N5 compares her new position with sonographers in another clinic who were not given responsibility for breaking bad news,

> N5: *Which must be an awful job for them … it must be hard, a lot of the times they can't say anything to them can they?*

Interviewer: *No*

N5: *Which I think is a good thing that we can, we're not leaving them.*

The nurses felt a need to be conscious of the effects of emotions on themselves and their patients and to work to manage these emotions effectively. In the following quote, N2 acknowledges that fertility work is difficult because of the emotional effects and suggests that a fertility nurse also has to have a stable personality to cope,

N2: *I think you have to be quite a stable personality to cope with the ups and downs. I think people can look at the fertility nurse and think 'nice clinic job, and like outpatients', which it is certainly not …*

Interviewer: *No.*

N2: *The highs and lows are probably more than anything I've ever worked in before.*

One way of coping is distancing one's own emotions from the patients'. N5 feels that the burden and effects of their emotions are sometimes too much to bear and suggests that infertile couples need to manage their emotions themselves.

Trying not to be too down about it but being honest. It's really the best thing to do but be positive about it as well if you can. Knowing you can't do anything and … they've got to accept responsibility for themselves, they're grown-ups at the end of the day. It's a big thing for them in their life and passing it back to them as well because it's hard for you then to accept all this responsibility for everybody.

The health care assistant (HCA) also found emotions were difficult to manage and felt that she had to manage her emotions in order to be the cheerful one amidst the 'bad news' in the clinic.

HCA: *Um, I just think it's because I'm not a medical person … that I'm not going to tell them the bad news. So I'm the one that's always sort of happy go lucky and try to keep them sort of … going in smiling. So I'm not going to be in a bad mood.*

In the following quote, the health care assistant seems to acknowledge that remaining cheerful and not being involved is difficult.

Interviewer: *Yeah, yeah, so what parts of the job do you find most satisfying?*

HCA: *Oh, um, the end result, to actually see the patient. Like at the birthday party literally [they] come running across to you, so happy that y'know they were told they would never have a child and at the end of the day you've gone against what nature has said and given them the end result …*

Interviewer: *Do you get lots of tears?*

HCA: *Um, mostly mine (laughs). You can't not get emotionally involved. You'd be a hard person if you didn't. You'd like to leave it all at home, or leave it all here, but you still do take some of it home with you, you can't not.*

Interpersonal factors

The data suggest that interpersonal factors such as support, interprofessional working and the internal milieu within the unit influence new nursing roles. These factors assisted nurses to develop new roles and undertake medical procedures.

> *There's an open culture. It's not like Consultant 1 is letting you do this and I'll do it whether I'm happy or not. They accept that the days where we were told what to do and you do it even if you don't agree, they're gone.* (N2)

Our field observations and interview data suggested that the new roles have led to more equal team dynamics in comparison to team dynamics in other areas. This collegial interprofessional working was viewed in a positive light and contributed to nurses' willingness to change roles and take on more responsibility.

> *I think the dynamics within the team itself is important because we all get on very well together. We're very different but we seem to gel and there aren't any tensions between us. We've all been in theatres and the way surgeons behave … we don't have that attitude and we're all on an equal level.* (N2)

The internal milieu of the clinic facilitated role change because nurses felt they were supported and that they had a real choice about undertaking new roles. The multiprofessional skills training introduced into the clinic suggests that training and supervision of new staff were taken seriously. These levels of support and training have led nurses to accept new roles and increased responsibility for performing medical tasks such as egg pickup. Our field notes show that there are a range of ways in which nurses now work which demonstrate an integration of new technical skills with caring skills.

> *Nurse C went to perform an egg pickup for Nurse G's patient. The couple had spent time with Nurse G who prepared them post consent and inserted the venflon and sedation. Nurse E assisted Nurse C with egg pickup and Nurse G focused on the couple.* (Field notes, 1.7.01)

We argue that each situation changes dynamics in medical procedures because of nurses' knowledge of both positions: that of the doctor or nurse performing the task and that of the nurse assisting the doctor and caring for the patient. N1 describes working and knowing each other as nurses in the following situation:

> *The main carer is the person who's taken the patient through from the waiting room because she's spent longer with that patient. Her role is to observe, watch, hold hands whereas the person who's operati[ng] can't do that, you can't do everything, you have to have an awareness of what's happening but of everything, what's happening in the lab, what the assistant needs to do, what the other nurse is doing, what the husband's doing … you have to have the whole picture. The nurse who's looking after the patient really has that as her main focus and while she concentrates on the task, her focus is the patient. We know how each other works and perhaps I can suggest something to the other nurse without them thinking 'I'm being told what to do', you know.*

Awareness of both positions enables the nurse undertaking the medical procedure to perform the procedure differently from a traditional nursing or medical position as N4 suggests in the following quote,

> Interviewer: *Do you feel the environment between doctor–nurse or nurse–nurse scenarios is different?*
> N4: *There is a difference in that they do the same job, just as well as each other. The nurses tend to talk more during the*

procedure. Explain to patients what they're doing. If somebody's jumping with pain, they tend to stop, give more sedation and then start again. I've noticed C1 does that now more often! (Laughs)

Changes in team dynamics were described as having led to a more relaxed atmosphere during the procedure as N4 describes,

The way we work there's always a third person in the room. There's a big overlap of roles and sometimes the doctor or nurse will point out to the patient and the partner the screen. There's a lot of three way traffic going on between the operator who is talking to the patient and the nurse assisting and it's not separation of roles at all. (N4)

Annandale *et al.* (1999) have previously suggested that nurses' traditional work orientates them to patients as a collective and is therefore task-based and fragmented. Allan (1999) has argued that nurses' work in fertility care is fragmented with the nurse taking a central role in organising the clinic rather than caring for individual patients. Our data suggests that these new nursing roles may have reduced fragmentation and increased continuity for nurses. Patients' views on these new roles were not elicited in the interviews and they appeared not to have been conscious of interpersonal factors. However, they noticed and stressed the importance of continuity, availability of 'their' nurse and bonding to the nurse allocated to them during their treatment cycles.

Socio-cultural factors: justifying changing roles

Socio-cultural factors

Socio-cultural factors which emerged in the data were the internal cultural milieu of the unit and the external milieu of medical and nursing fertility practice. A significant feature of the internal milieu in the unit was the relationship between the past and present medical directors and the nurses. This relationship and the support they had received from these two consultants was commented on by all the nurses as being significant in their decision to undertake and develop an advanced role,

Consultant 2 was radical and didn't care what the establishment said. He was independent. He was very good at building

people up, empowering them. He was very good, empowering us to make our own decisions but he was there if we needed him. He trusted us enough to get on with it. (N1)

This encouragement was based on trust within the clinic and it was observed that this trust was absent outside the clinic,

There's a lack of trust that nurses experience from doctors because they don't think nurses have the academic background ... some doctors dismiss nurses as not understanding. (N1)

The nurses and the doctor interviewed were aware that, while they might view developing the nursing role as a natural extension of specialist practice, others outside in the fertility field did not. They perceived the external nursing and medical milieu as hostile to, and distrustful of, new nursing roles.

Whenever I do presentations on my role, you get either people saying 'Ooh, that's really good but we're not allowed to do that' or they feel very threatened by it because they think people will expect them to do the same. Initially when Consultant 2 asked me to do pickup, I said no because the climate [outside] wasn't right. (N1)

There were two aspects of the data which surprised us. The first was the extent to which the doctor also felt the need to 'keep quiet' about these role changes and the multi-professional teaching programme she had begun to develop. The second was the fragility of the role change and how, in certain situations, for example working with locum doctors, nurses retreated from their new roles. The data suggests that professional communities can exert a pressure, perhaps unseen, around issues related to changing roles and consequently relationships between doctors and nurses. As Consultant 1 says:

I think it's well known within the fertility nursing community. It's not well recognised within the medical community. I certainly don't hide the fact but I don't go out of my way to talk about it. I think probably because of an unconscious anxiety that many clinicians would be unhappy with what they would see as nurses doing essentially doctors' roles.

The experience of these staff suggests that the external milieu of the fertility 'world', the professional community, has been experienced as hostile and medically dominated. Whereas the internal milieu of the clinic has been experienced by staff as protective, nurturing and willing to take risks. The meanings given to these new nursing roles by the nurses and the influences on their development are now discussed in relation to the literature and the unexplored consequences of government thinking around changing roles in health care.

Discussion

This group of nurses believed that the changes in nursing practice increased the nurse's ability to know and, therefore, provide continuity of care for the infertile couple. This was their moral justification for the role changes. However, continuity of care brought about by continuity of carer did not mean a change in the knowing between nurse and patients. The nurses believed that 'knowing a patient' contained a distance and was a professional knowing rather than an intimate form of knowing.

One of the significant aspects of the data is how the nature of the task shaped the nature of the nurse–patient relationship and the forms of intimacy and knowing which were developed. The investigation and treatment cycle for infertile patients is highly intimate and intrusive not only because it deals with intimate areas of the body for both men and women (Meerabeau 1999; Allan 2001). It also deals with an intimate ontological area of being a man or woman who is unable to conceive and bear children (Franklin 1990; Pines 1993; Raphael-Leff 1991; Christie 1998). Nurses in this study recognised that intimacy was 'forced' because patients had to consent to intrusive procedures to have any success of conception. They also recognised that the degree of intimacy in the physical sense shaped and restricted, for some patients, the level of intimacy in the social sense. The intimacy was focused quite specifically on a narrow area of the patient's lives and did not generally go beyond this area. In this way, the task and the forced nature of the intimacy seemed to demand a nurse–patient relationship which was more distanced rather than intimate (Girard 1988; Meerabeau 1999).

However, nurses did not feel that their relationships with infertile patients were dominated by medical tasks. They argued that their roles could improve continuity for patients and hence knowing, intimacy and support for patients. They quite clearly justified their roles in terms of developing patient-centred care (RCN 2003). The critiques of new nursing roles have argued that nursing roles which undertake medical tasks assume a hierarchy of knowledge with medical knowledge being at the top of the hierarchy (RCN 2003). The data suggests that this is rejected by this group of nurses who see their roles as developing from patient need rather than being imposed by management or from a desire for increased pay or status. The data also suggest that nurses create a 'narrative' to justify their new nursing roles and we argue that they felt the need to construct these narratives because of their experiences of being criticised by both their nursing and medical colleagues. The narratives contain the justification and explanation for the changes in working practices as well as their motives for changing their practice. Their motivations appeared to be an important factor in shaping whether an individual nurse would take on a new role.

Government policy suggests that developing new roles and flexibility in teams will assist in modernising the NHS (NHS Plan DH 2000). The RCN (2003:7) has stated that ' teamwork health care should be provided by a team with different but complementary skills where it does not matter who within the team provides care'. The work undertaken to develop the new roles in this clinic is an example of such flexible work practices where professional barriers are broken down and the needs of the patient are placed at the centre of care delivery. Such role changes and partnerships need to be analysed critically because they raise some interesting questions about the nature, meaning and context of medical and nursing tasks as well as the experience of inter-professional working.

This data shows that while the definitions of medical and nursing tasks may change, the nature of the task remains unchanged, that is, a procedure remains intrinsically the same whoever is performing it providing the person performing the task is competent. In the data it appears that the context of the task and the continuity of carer rather than the task itself is important to patients and staff. The patients' emphasis on continuity of carer implies that the context of continuity of carer becomes imbued with meaning for patients over the concerns of professional boundaries or flexible working. It is also suggested that while the task remains the same, the manner of its delivery is important to patients. This would confirm other studies in primary care, for example Ashburner *et al.* 1997, which suggest that patients prefer nurse consultations even where there are no measurable differences in outcomes.

In addition, the data shows that these changes may enhance care as patients benefit from advanced knowledge from doctors in the most complex cases and continuity of carer from nurses under supervision from doctors. In these new roles where there are new lines of responsibility and accountability underpinned by clinical governance, the different values, attitudes and skills of each profession are arguably utilised to the patient's best advantage.

The data does not illuminate the consequences of these new roles for doctors as they become less directly involved in routine medical tasks and develop a more supervisory role. In this supervisory capacity, two potential types of practice are possible. Either the medical role may become less orientated to individuals as the doctor gives attention to the clinic as a whole which would give them less continuity. Or the doctor focuses on the more complex patients and remains orientated to such individual patients. This would appear to confirm Annandale *et al.*'s findings (1999) that the potential for continuity in the medical role stems from their ability to focus on the patient rather than groups of patients. The data suggests that the fragmented task is reduced for the nurse as she becomes a continuous figure for the infertile couple in performing advanced roles. And for doctors, the fragmented task may not be increased if they remain engaged with individual patients.

Conclusions

I have argued that new nursing roles are changing staff's attitudes to interprofessional working by subtly redrawing the boundaries between professions in the AR clinics in areas such as skills, knowledge, autonomy and responsibility. The evidence for the changes to these boundaries has been presented in the data. An important aspect of these changes is the difference between the internal world of the clinic which has supported these changes and the external world of fertility which has seen these changes as threatening.

The nurses and the doctor in this unit were able to explain their motivations for such changes through their narratives which justified their new roles. The justifications for their new roles were based on the improved continuity in their relationships with patients, which led to them 'knowing' patients and providing a different type of care to doctors. Some of the data adds to previous work in this area of knowing and intimacy by focusing on how nurse–patient relationships are shaped by the nature and location of the nursing task and the patient's condition. We argue that understanding nurses' motives for developing higher levels of practice develops the profession's understanding of the consequences of new nursing roles for patients, nurses and their medical colleagues.

What is clear from the data is that nurses undertake role development (advanced roles) because it meets the aim of nursing, which for these nurses is delivering caring and enhancing the caring relationship. Working with their own and patients' emotions is central to this relationship. In the final chapter these themes of caring and emotions are drawn together to discuss the implications of developing such advanced nursing roles in the current political and economic climates.

Reflection:

Do the changes in health care delivery make advanced nursing roles inevitable?

Chapter 9
Conclusions

The underlying assumption in this book is that caring and working with emotions are the key aims of any nursing role whether in fertility or women's health. I have described how, in both advanced fertility nursing roles and more traditional nursing roles, the central focus has been caring for patients. Working with emotions in a caring role is not easily achieved however. Hence, I have described caring behaviours which involved working with emotions, sometimes unconsciously and sometime consciously; and at times unsuccessfully and at others, more successfully. In this chapter attention is drawn to:

- some trends in ARTs and wider health care policy generally, which threaten nurses' ability to focus on care and emotions, whether in traditional or advanced roles

- a broader discussion of women's health to consider the nature of advanced nursing practice in the context of pressure on resources for health care funding (Temmink *et al.* 2000; Allan 2007b).

- the complexity of nursing role development and the argument for nursing to remain open to many different forms, to meet the needs of the patient rather than constrain it to 'fit' a particular professional ideology.

Current trends in ARTs in the UK

Current trends

The use of ARTs is increasing in the UK (HFEA 2008) with quite subtle changes in the demographics of couples seeking ARTs (they tend to be older) and in the causes of infertility (male infertility is now the largest cause of infertility).

Transport IVF

There is a trend to manage patients using transport IVF and satellite clinics (Qureshi *et al.* 1997; Brinsden 2003). Satellite IVF is where the assessment, drug therapy and monitoring take place at the secondary (satellite) centre but the egg retrieval, embryology and embryo replacement are all carried out at the primary (licensed) centre. This system can reduce travel time for patients and more of the interventions can be undertaken closer to home.

At the same time AR clinics and their clinical directors have facilitated the types of advanced nursing roles described in this book (Corrigan 1996; Birch 2001). It is interesting that the nurses in study 2 did not operate a transport IVF system; i.e. patients visited the AR clinics for their entire treatment protocol and consequently were able to maintain contact with the same nurse during each cycle. In fact, patients would choose not to have a particular cycle if they knew their nurse would be on holiday at that time.

I have argued elsewhere (Allan *et al.* in press) that the introduction of technology and managing patients at a distance (which is essentially what transport IVF is) may threaten the advanced roles I have described in this book. Increasing use of technologies to manage patients on care pathways at a distance from the central AR clinics may erode the support provided by the clinic and offer less continuity of care. But equally such systems may offer less disruption to patients' lives and benefit women in other ways. Van Dongen & Elema (2001) argue that technologies may alter patient and nurse satisfaction because they interfere with touch and caring practices. However, as IVF and other ARTs become increasingly routinised, transport IVF may offer women ways to control the IVF process (Allan *et al.* in press) because they can choose where to have their bloods and ultrasound scans done and by whom. They can also control the form of relationship and intimacy they wish to develop within each AR clinic.

While transport IVF may offer choice, the control permitted by distance may produce more ambivalence for women because the lack of intimacy, the possibilities of chaperoning and the 'containment' of the liminal space in the clinic suggested in this book are not possible. It appears that both the clinic and transport IVF offer possibilities for choice and control; on the one hand transport IVF offers possibilities for negotiating embodiment while at the same time restricting the potential for intimacy and care. The AR clinics offer the possibility of intimacy albeit negotiated and distant while reinforcing the biomedical objectification of the body.

Funding of fertility treatments

Trends in forms of care delivery in AR clinics are also fundamentally shaped by medical control and the pursuit of profits in privately funded health care sectors which provide the majority of ARTs. In fact, 85% of ARTs are paid for by patients themselves (Brinsden 2003). Infertility as a medicalised disease offers fertile ground for competing professional interests. As the funding of fertility treatments in the UK continues to be predominantly a matter for the private health care sector, clinics will be under pressure to increase profits and respond to demands. One possible demand is suggested in the HFEA's data analysis of the register's statistics (2008) which suggest that cumulative live birth rates are improved by the number of cycles delivered. In addition, age and fertility rate do not seem to be affected; that is, age does not affect fertilisation rate although it does affect live birth rate. This may present a demand for increased numbers of cycles in a population of couples who are already ageing when they begin their ART journey.

These demands will occur in the context of staff and skills shortages (DH 2000; 2001; 2002) and inequalities in NHS provision of fertility treatments (BFS 2006). One of the drivers for fertility nursing role development in the UK has been the shortage of skilled, trained specialist staff to respond to an increasing demand for ARTs. Fertility nurses have been able to argue that specialist or advanced nursing knowledge provides safe and efficient care (Barber *et al.* 1996; Birch 2001) and in some cases, that outcomes can be improved if care is delivered by nurses rather than non-specialist medical staff. The question is whether British nursing will be able to retain these roles which have caring as their focus under these pressures. As for the traditional roles described in Chapter 4, I fear we have already lost the argument to retain these as Bradshaw argued in 2000. The data I have presented in this book shows how similar these two forms of roles are as they retain a key focus on caring and emotions.

Managing intimacy and emotions

What do we mean by advanced roles?

In a review of British ethnographic studies published between 1993 and 2003 which explore what nurses do, Allen (2004) has argued that nurses' work falls into the following functions:

- managing multiple agendas and occupational groups
- circulating patients (or managing patient journeys)
- managing personalised care in organisations which tend to standardise care
- managing the work of others (supporting doctors mainly)
- mediating occupational boundaries (plugging the gaps and working flexibly to ensure patients are cared for)
- being central to communication systems so that patients are informed
- recording nursing activity
- prioritising care and rationing resources.

Allen (2004) concludes from her review that nursing 'has little to gain by continuing to pursue an agenda of holistic care based on emotional intimacy' (2004:280). She argues that actually nurses manage the tensions inherent in any health care system which concern aspirations to individualised care on the one hand and standardised routines on the other. And she concludes that nurses need to be up front that what they do is to manage these tensions through the functions listed above. I would agree with this and say that what I describe as practical caring encompasses these functions and is highly skilled and has at heart the goal of supporting patients by managing the tensions Allen highlights in the health care system. At present, as I have argued elsewhere, there is a rhetorical claim to a certain form of caring, therapeutic caring, which is simply not evidence based (Luker 1997; Bradshaw 2000; Allen 2004; Allan 2007b). However nursing is something more as my data demonstrates – nurses acknowledge (at times and when supported to do so) and work with emotions both within patients, staff and the organisation itself (as discussed in Chapter 2).

On reviewing the data from both studies while writing this book, it seems to me that nurses working in the more traditional roles in study 1 used complex caring skills to work with the emotions evoked in practice; in doing so, they were unsupported and largely unreflective during everyday practice. However during the interviews for the study they were reflective and willing to explore how they were affected by the emotional tensions and stresses of their clinical work. Their primary focus was on running the clinic and supporting patients and doctors even when these aims were in tension. In study 2, the nurses working in advanced roles were working with the same approach as those nurses in study 1, namely to support patients. To this end, they undertook these new roles. Central to both these ways of nursing was a concern with caring as the primary focus of nursing and managing emotions which they recognised (at times unconsciously and at other times, consciously) was a difficulty for them and their patients.

Advanced practice in women's health

Advanced practice

From this data, to define advanced roles in women's health more widely I would argue that the following is a key aim: caring and working with patients' and their own emotions effectively.

Of course, in many situations, nurses do not deliver care directly (Luker 1997; Bradshaw 2000; Allen 2004; Allan 2007b). I would argue that even where nurses are unable to retain everyday delivery of care, they need to supervise and work with those who provide this care to ensure that skilled, knowledgeable caring, what I term practical caring, remains at the heart of nursing. The moral justification and the logical rationale for this position is because (as Menzies [1970] and Taylor [personal communication] have argued), working with emotions in a caring relationship has always been and will continue to be at the heart of health care.

Having established caring and working with emotions as the key aim of an advanced nursing role, I would then build on Daly & Carnwell's (2003) framework along with the UKCC's (1996) competencies to include a:

- focus on role extension (i.e. tasks possibly from other disciplines) which make the nursing role more effective as in the case of advanced fertility nursing roles I have described;
- focus on role expansion (elements which build on specialist nursing knowledge);

- focus on role development (higher levels of clinical autonomy) which meet patient need.

The transgressive nature of caring in nursing

Transgressive nature of caring

I have argued in this book that re-asserting the value of caring in nursing practice through the role of chaperoning, hovering or being there for instance, might be seen as transgressive or challenging to current professional models of nursing practice because these roles appear to hark back to a former model of nursing. These former ways of nursing are negatively portrayed as old-fashioned and traditional (Luker 1997) in the context of a modernising NHS which seeks to change and educate to meet changing health care needs (DH 2000). In reflecting on changes in nursing systems from traditional to new nursing, Luker points out, 'change has been driven forward by evangelical zeal, based on the belief that new was better than old' (1997:263). These traditional forms of nursing are understood to be merely supportive to doctors but actually the data show that they facilitate nurses to assist, support and respond to patients through being present and reacting to their distress in a thoughtful way. It is the invisibility of these forms of caring work which has proved problematic in the policy debates about modernising the health services (as Allen [2004] also points out). The strength of this data is that it makes visible what has been rendered invisible and in so doing, make it seem transgressive because it appears, nursing is more than just caring (Bradshaw 2000) and can be more than a claim to care (Allan 2007b). The transgressive nature of these roles is made more striking in the context of the drive for efficiency in the NHS as skilled caring work is not necessarily efficient (Luker 1997).

But surely, advanced roles meet the requirements of the modern NHS? We already know from other empirical data (Ashburner *et al.* 1997) that advanced roles such as nurse practitioners do not prove cost effective. And as Land *et al.* (1996) argue, practitioners may develop roles without any appropriate preparation, holistic integration or clinical autonomy which makes them difficult to support, evaluate and educate for. The findings from study 2 (presented in Chapter 8) confirm that advanced nursing roles do not always develop in the ways intended by policy. In undertaking advanced roles, nurses retain caring as the key focus of their role and appear to need a moral narrative to justify their advanced roles. I believe that these moral narratives are necessary for nurses because these roles appear transgressive in the three ways discussed below:

1. Working with emotions, not emotional closeness

These roles challenge influential theories of caring in nursing (Luker 1997) which assert that emotional closeness or intimacy is the goal of professional nursing practice. This data suggests that working with emotions is possible but does not always result (nor should it) in close, intimate relationships. These relationships can be therapeutic without closeness and are valued by patients.

2. Caring as part of the advanced nursing role

Advanced roles challenge models of workforce development based on role substitution (medical roles for nursing roles) because they reassert caring as part of an advanced nursing role. Luker (1997) argues that caring by nurses is seen as too expensive and inefficient for the modernising, efficient NHS which is why substituting assistants for trained nurses is popular in policy terms; but this data shows that nurses and patients do not agree. As can be seen in Chapter 8, there has always been a concern that nursing role development retains a focus on caring (Manley 1997) even though the DH (1994) confirmed that the role of nurse includes caring as a core element which underpins other functions:

- coordination
- teaching
- developing and maintaining programmes of care
- technical expertise
- concern for those who are ill and those currently well
- special responsibility for the frail and vulnerable.

In addition to challenging models of professional development which do not place so much emphasis on caring, this data challenges the new nursing where caring as a therapeutic relationship was very much at the heart of nursing. These nurses are quite clear that such close, intimate forms of relationships are unrealistic and not appropriate.

Luker (1997) and Bradshaw (2000) have both argued for nurses to retain control over, and practice, caring. These roles suggest that this is possible in specialised fields such as fertility nursing. The nurses were able to retain management over delegation of caring tasks to HCAs as well as keep caring as the key focus of role development. The moral narratives could be how they did this. As one nurse asked, how can this role development be justified? Will it benefit my patient?

3. The value of gendered caring

The data also asserts gendered caring, i.e. that being a woman in caring for an infertile woman going through ARTs is important for patients. Current writing on the gender relations in nursing and the gendered nature of nursing suggest that the male and female are seen as essentially differentiated and the female is devalued (Porter 1992; Evans 1996). On top of this differentiation, another exists which is built on gender namely, skills (masculine) and caring (feminine) (Porter 1992). However, in a study into gynaecology nursing, Bolton (2005) explored female gynaecology nurses' experiences of doing women's work, i.e. gynaecology nursing and found that these nurses valued 'women's job carrying out women's work'. In contrast to previous writing, gendered nursing was valued as a strength of nursing. The nurses valued doing women's work because they felt men could not work in gynaecology as they did not have the skills or knowledge and would not be able to manage the distress and 'dirty' work of miscarriages and menstruation. They resented male gynaecologists who they saw as trespassing in women's work. Far from seeing themselves as having less valuable knowledge than men, they saw themselves as strong, professional women. Bolton (2005) argues that the association between women, mothering, caring and nursing was rejected during the later half of the 20th century. This is because the association was generally seen as an essentialist argument, i.e. one that reinforces women's subordination to men in a patriarchal hierarchy. Women's special skills and knowledge were seen as less valuable than scientific knowledge and evidence-based practice and this was thought to create a negative situation for women nurses. Women's knowledge and skills were often rejected by women because it was seen to be based on unfixed gender identities and characteristics which are presumed meaningful across social class and race.

I have suggested here that reasserting the value of caring and working with emotions in nursing practice might be seen as transgressive to current professional models of nursing practice and in the context of a modernising NHS. However, based on this data, I think that nursing roles (whether they are advanced, specialist or just qualified) which locate caring and working with emotions at the heart of nursing could address patients' needs (Fabricius 1991a; 1991b).

Nursing role development: Implications for practice

Nursing role development

It may seem as if I have outlined an inexorable progress to advanced nursing roles where caring and attention to emotions become difficult if not impossible. I do not see this necessarily happening and believe that nurses control and shape the forms of advanced nursing roles which emerge in the future. I do not say this will be easy, merely that it is possible. I think as a profession, the Royal College of Nursing's Dignity campaign is an example of keeping caring at the forefront of both patients' and policy makers' agendas. However, as the nurses in study 2 found, each nurse needs to influence the exact scope of any advanced role they take on. They may need to draw upon other nurses for support in managing resistance to exerting control over the exact nature of these roles. Support can be found at unit level, through interdisciplinary relationships and at an organisational level. Outside the employing organisation, there is support available such as the Association of Psychosexual Nurses and linking with like-minded nurses who are keen to keep caring and emotions at the forefront of practice.

Final thoughts
Given this data, it seems to me that the complexity of nursing requires a complex role development which is reflexive. It needs to remain open to many different forms of nursing to meet the needs of the patient rather than constrain it to 'fit' a particular professional ideology.

References

Aldridge, M. (1994) Unlimited liability? Emotional labour in nursing and social work, *Journal of Advanced Nursing,* **20**(4): 722–728.

Allan, H.T. (1999) *Sister will see you now: Managing emotions in AR clinics*. PhD Thesis, University of Manchester.

Allan, H.T. (2001) Nursing the clinic and managing emotions in a fertility unit: Findings from an ethnographic study. *Nursing Inquiry* **8**: 51–60.

Allan, H.T. (2001) A 'good enough' nurse: supporting patients in a fertility unit. *Human Fertility* **4**: 18–23.

Allan, H.T. (2002) Nursing the clinic, being there, hovering: Ways of caring in a British fertility unit. *Journal of Advanced Nursing* **38**(1): 86–93.

Allan, H.T. (2005) Gender and embodiment in nursing: the role of the female chaperone in the AR clinics. *Nursing Inquiry* **12**(3): 175–183

Allan, H.T. (2007a) Liminality and the experience of infertility: the role of the clinic in creating a liminal space. *Nursing Inquiry* **14**(2): 132–139

Allan, H.T. (2007b) The rhetoric of caring and the recruitment of overseas nurses: the social reproduction of a care gap. *Journal of Clinical Nursing Special Edition* **16**(12): 2204–2212

Allan, H.T. & Barber, D. (2004) Nothing out of the ordinary: Advanced fertility nursing practice. *Human Fertility* **7**: 277–284.

Allan, H.T. & Barber, D. (2005) Emotion boundary work in advanced fertility nursing roles. *Nursing Ethics* **12**(4): 391–400.

Allan, H.T., De Lacey, S. & Payne, D. (forthcoming) The socio-cultural context of assisted reproductive technologies: the shaping of routine practices. *Nursing Inquiry.*

Allen, D. (2004) Re-reading nursing and re-writing practice: towards an empirically based reformulation of the nursing mandate. *Nursing Inquiry* **11**: 271–283.

Anderson, E.R. (1973) *The Role of the Nurse*, London: RCN/National Council of Nurses of the United Kingdom.

Annandale, E., Clark, J. & Allen, E. (1999) Interprofessional working: an ethnographic case study of emergency health care. *Journal of Interprofessional Care* **13**(2):139–150.

Armstrong-Esther, C. A., Browne, K.D. and McAfee, J.G. (1994) Elderly patients: still clean and sitting quietly *Journal of Advanced Nursing* **19**(2): 264–271.

Ashburner, L., Birch, K., Latimer, J. & Scrivens, E. (1997) *Nurse Practitioners in Primary Care*. Centre for Health Planning and Management, Keele University, Staffs.

Ashworth, P.D., Longmate, M.A. & Morrison, P. (1992) Patient participation: its meaning and significance in the context of caring. *Journal of Advanced Nursing* **17**(12): 1430–1439.

Atkinson, P. (1993) *Medical Talk and Medical Work*. London: Routledge.

Badcock, C. (1992) *Essential Freud*. Second edition. Oxford: Blackwell.

Balint, E. (1964) *The Doctor, his Patient and the Illness*. London: Pitman Medical.

Barber, D., Egan, D., Ross, C., Evans, B. & Barlow, D. (1996) Nurses performing embryo transfer: Successful outcome of IVF. *Human Reproduction* **11**: 105–108.

Barber, P. (1991) Caring: the nature of the therapeutic relationship. In: Jolley, M., Perry, A. (editors) *Nursing: a knowledge base for practice*. London: Edward Arnold: 230–270.

Barber, D. (1997) Research into the role of fertility nurses for the development of guidelines for clinical practice. *Human Reproduction* **12**: 195–197.

Managing intimacy and emotions

Barnes, E., Griffiths, P., Ord, J., & Wells, D. (1998) (editors) *Face to Face with Distress: The Professional Use of Self in Psychosocial Care*. Oxford: Butterworth Heinemann.

Becker, G. (1999) *Disrupted Lives. How people create meaning in a chaotic world*. London: University of California Press.

Benner, P. & Wrubel, J. (1989) *The Primacy of Caring*. Menlo Park, CA: Addison Wesley.

Bennet, S. & Templeton, A. (1995) The epidemiology of infertility. In *Infertility Nursing and Caring*, Meerabeau, L & Denton, J. (editors) 42–55. London: Scutari Press.

Bignell, C.J. (1999) Chaperones for genital examination. *British Medical Journal* **319**: 137–138.

Birch, H. (2001) The extended role of the nurse – opportunity or threat? *Human Fertility* **4**(3): 138–144

Bloch, M. & Parry, J. (1982) *Death and the Regeneration of Life*. Cambridge: Cambridge University Press.

Bolton, S. (2005) Women's work, dirty work: the gynaecology nurse as 'other'. *Gender, Work and Organisation* **12**(2): 169–186

Boivin, J. (2008) Is there too much emphasis on psychosocial counseling for infertile patients? *Journal of Assisted Reproduction and Genetic*. **14**(4): 184–186.

Bowden, P.L. (1995) The ethics of nursing care and the ethic of care. *Nursing Inquiry* **2**(10): 10–21.

Bowden, P.L. (1997) *Caring: gender-sensitive ethics*. London: Routledge.

Boyle, M. & McEvoy, J. (1998) Putting abortion in its social context: Northern Irish women's experiences of abortion in England. *Health: An International Journal for the Social Study of Health, Illness and Medicine* **2**: 283–304.

Bradshaw, A. (1995) What are nurses doing to patients? A review of theories of nursing past and present. *Journal of Clinical Nursing* **4**(2): 81–92

Bradshaw, A. (2000) Competence and British nursing: a view from history. *Journal of Clinical Nursing* **9**(3): 321–329.

Branaman, A. (1997) Goffman's Social Theory. In Lemert, C. & Branaman, A. (editors) *The Goffman Reader*. Oxford:Blackwell Publishers Inc.

Brewin, T.B. (1993) How much ethics is needed to make a good doctor? *Lancet*. **341**, Nov.16: 161–163.

Brilowski, G.A. & Wendler, M.C. (2005) An evolutionary concept analysis of caring. *Journal of Advanced Nursing* **50**(6): 641–650.

Bringhenti, F., Martinelli, F., Ardenti, R. & Battista La Sala, G. (1997) Psychological adjustment of infertile women entering IVF treatment: differentiating aspects and influencing factors. *Acta Obstetricia et Gynecologica Scandinavica* **76**(5): 431–437.

Brinsden, P. (2003) Models for future delivery of care in infertility: the role of the private sector. *Human Fertility* **6**(2): Supplement 1: S25–27.

British Fertility Society (2006) *Survey of NHS fertility treatment across England shows inequalities; fertility doctors set out social criteria access to treatment*. Media Release. http://www.britishfertilitysociety.org.uk/news/documents/SocialCriteriaAndNICEImplementation30Aug06.doc (Accessed 31/07/08).

British Infertility Counselling Association. (2005) BICA's response to the Department of Health's consultation 'Review of the Human Fertilisation and Embryology Act'. *Journal of Fertility Counselling* **12**: 11–19.

Bryant-Lukosius, D., DiCenso, A., Browne, G. & Pinelli, J. (2004) Advanced practice nursing roles: development, implementation and evaluation. *Journal of Advanced Nursing* **48**(5): 519–529.

Burawoy, M. (1998) The extended case study method. *Sociological Theory* **16**(1): 4–33.

Cannell, F. (1990) Concepts of parenthood: the Warnock report, the Gillick debate and modern myths. *American Ethnologist* **17**: 667–686.

Carpenter, M. (1993) The subordination of nurses in healthcare: towards a social divisions approach. In Riska, E. & Wegar, K. (editors) *Gender Work and Medicine: Women and the Medical Division of Labour* 109–126. London: Sage Publications.

Carr, E.K., Friedman, T. Lannon, B. & Sharp, B. (1990) The study of psychological factors in couples receiving artificial insemination by donor: a discussion of methodological difficulties. *Journal of Advanced Nursing* **15**(8): 906–910.

Champion, V. Austin, J. and Tzeng, O.C.S. (1987) Cross cultural comparison of images of nurses and physicians. *International Nursing Review*, **34**(2): 43–48.

Christianson, C. (1986) Support groups for infertile patients. *Journal of Obstetric, Gynecologic and Neonatal Nursing* **15**(4): 293–296.

Chodorow, N. (1974) Family structure and feminine personality. In Rosaldo, M. X. & Lamphere, L. (editors), *Women, culture and society.* Stanford University Press 43–66.

Chodorow, N. (1989) *Feminism and psychoanalytic theory.* London: Yale University Press.

Chodorow, N. (2003) Too late: Ambivalence about motherhood, choice and time. In Alcira, M.A. (editor), *Studies on Femininity.* London: Karnac Books 27–40.

Christie, G. (1998) Some socio-cultural and psychological aspects of infertility. *Human Reproduction* **13**: 232–241.

Clarke, J.B. & Wheeler, S.J. (1992) A view of the phenomenon of caring in nursing practice. *Journal of Advanced Nursing* **17**(11): 1283–1290.

Clifford, C. (1995) Caring: fitting the concept to nursing practice. *Journal of Clinical Nursing* **4**(1): 37–41.

Clifford, D. (1998) Psychosexual awareness in everyday nursing *Nursing Standard* **12**(39):42–45.

Clifford, D., Rutter, M. & Selby, J. (2000) *Caring for Sexuality in Health and Illness.* Wells, D. (editor) London: Churchill Livingstone.

Colliere, M.F. (1986) Invisible care and invisible women as health care providers. *International Journal of Nursing Studies* **23**(2): 95–112.

Connell, R.W. (1987) *Gender, Power and Society, the Person and Sexual Politics.* Cambridge: Polity Press.

Coombs, M. & Ersser, S. (2004) Medical hegemony in decision-making – a barrier to interdisciplinary working in intensive care? *Journal of Advanced Nursing* **46**(3): 245–252.

Corrigan, L. (1996) The roles and expectations of the infertility nurse practitioner and the scope for extended nursing practice. *Journal of British Fertility* **1**(1): 61–64.

Cousineau, T.M., Green, T.C., Corsini, E.A., Barbard, T., Seibring, A.R. & Domar, A.D. (2006) Development and validation of the infertility self-efficacy scale. *Fertility & Sterility* **85**(6): 1684–1696.

Craib, I. (1995) Some comments on the sociology of emotions. *Sociology* **29**: 151–58.

Croft, M. (1999) Chaperones should always be present. *British Medical Journal* **319**: 1266.

Crossley, N. (1996) Merleau-Ponty, the elusive body and carnal sociology. *Body and Society* **1**: 43–63.

Csordas, T.J. 1994. *Embodiment and Experience, the Existential Ground of Culture and Self.* Cambridge: University of Cambridge.

Czarniawska, B. & Mazza, C. (2003) Consulting as a liminal space. *Human Relations* **56**: 267–290.

de Lacey, S. (2002) IVF as a lottery or investment: Contesting metaphors in discourses of infertility. *Nursing Inquiry* **9**: 43–51.

de Raeve, L. (2002) The modification of emotional responses: a problem for trust in nurse-patient relationships? *Nursing Ethics* **9**: 465–471.

Dalley, G. (1995) *Ideologies of Caring: Rethinking Community and Collectivism*, (2nd Edition). Basingstoke: Macmillan (in Association with the Centre for Policy on Ageing).

Managing intimacy and emotions

Daly, W.M. & Carnwell, R. (2003) Nursing roles and levels of practice: a framework for differentiating between elementary, specialist and advancing nursing practice. *Journal of Clinical Nursing* **12**:158–167.

Daniels, A.K. (1987) Invisible work. *Social Problems* **34**(5): 403–413.

Darwin, C. (1955) *The Expression of Emotions in Man and Animals*. New York: Philosophical Library.

Davies, C. (1995) *Gender and the Professional Predicament of Nursing*. Buckingham: Open University Press.

Davies, K. (2003) The body and doing gender: The relations between doctors and nurses in hospital work. *Sociology of Health and Illness* **25**: 720–742.

Davis, D.C. and Dearman, C.N. (1991) Coping Strategies of Infertile Women. *Journal of Obstetric, Gynecologic and Neonatal Nursing* **20**(3): 221–228.

Department of Health (1994) *The Challenges for Nursing and Midwifery in the 21st Century*. London: HMSO.

Department of Health (1997a) *Taking the Temperature of the New Deal: an evaluation of the New Deal on junior doctor's hours and its implications for flexible working practices*. London: HMSO.

Department of Health (1997b) *The new NHS: modern, dependable*. London: HMSO.

Department of Health (1999) *Agenda for Change: Modernising the NHS pay system*. London: HMSO.

Department of Health (2000) *The NHS Plan*. London: HMSO

Department of Health (2001) *Doctors for the Future: Standing Medical Committee advice* (6/2001). http://www.dh.gov.uk/en/Publicationsandstatistics/Publications/PublicationsPolicyAndGuidance. (Accessed 31/07/08).

Department of Health (2002) *Creative Solutions to meeting clinical workforce shortfalls in the NHS: joint advice from the Standing Medical Advisory Committee and Standing Nursing and Midwifery Advisory Committee* (2002). http://www.dh.gov.uk/en/Publicationsandstatistics/Publications/PublicationsPolicyAndGuidance. (Accessed 31/07/08).

Department of Health (2003) *Guidance on Tackling Junior Doctors' Hours*. London: HMSO.

Department of Health (2005) *Review of the Human Fertilisation and Embryology Act*. London: HMSO.

Department of Health (2006) *Modernising Nursing Careers – setting the direction*. London: HMSO.

Department of Health (2007) *NHS Direct Interactive*. London: HMSO.

Department of Health (2008) *Towards a Framework for Post-registration Nursing Careers: a national consultation*. London: HMSO.

Deutsch, H. (1944) *The Psychology of Women, Volume 1: Girlhood*. New York: Grune & Stratton.

Deutsch, H. (1945) *The Psychology of Women, Volume 2: Motherhood*. New York: Grune & Stratton.

Dewey, J. (1922) *Human Nature and Conduct: an introduction to social psychology*. New York: Holt.

Douglas, M. (1966) *Purity and Danger*. London: Routledge.

Doyal, L. editor (1998) *Women and the Health Services*. Buckingham: Open University Press.

Duncombe, J. & Marsden, D. (1993) Love and intimacy: the gender division of emotion and 'emotion work'. *Sociology* **27**: 221–242.

Dunlop, M. (1986) Is a science of caring possible? *Journal of Advanced Nursing.* **11**(6): 661–670.

Editorial (2000) RCN guidelines on chaperoning. *Nursing Standard* **14**: 10.

Elder, A. and Samuel, O. (editors) (1987) *'While I'm here, doctor'. A study of the doctor-patient relationship*. London: Tavistock Publications Ltd.

English, V. (1995) The role of the Human Fertilisation and Embryology Authority. In *Infertility Nursing and Caring*, Meerabeau, L. & Denton, J. (editors) London: Scutari Press 156–167.

Ersser, S. (1991) A search for the therapeutic dimensions of nurse-patient interaction. In McMahon, R. & Pearson, A. (editors) *Nursing as Therapy*. London: Chapman-Hall: 43–84.

Ersser, S. (1997) *Nursing as a therapeutic activity, an ethnography*, Aldershot: Avebury.

Espeland, W. (1984) Blood and money: Exploiting the embodied self. In *The Existential Self in Society*, Kotarba, J. and Fontana, A. (editors) Chicago: University of Chicago Press 67–98.

Erskine, A. and Judd, D. (editors) (1994) *The Imaginative Body, Psychodynamic Therapy in Health Care*, London: Whurr Publishers Ltd.

Ettore, E. (1998) Review article: Re-shaping the space between bodies and culture: Embodying the biomedicalised body. *Sociology of Health and Illness* **20**: 548–55.

Eugster, A. & Vingerhoets, A.J.J.M. (1999) Psychological aspects of in vitro fertilisation: a review. *Social Science and Medicine* **48**(5): 575–589.

Evans, J. (1996) Men in nursing: issues of gender segregation and hidden advantage. *Journal of Advanced Nursing* **26**(2): 226–231.

Fabricius, J. (1991a) Learning to work with feelings — a psychodynamic understanding and small group work with junior student nurses. *Nurse Education Today* **11**: 134–142.

Fabricius, J. (1991b) Running on the spot or can nursing really change? *Psychoanalytic Psychotherapy* **5**: 97–108.

Fabricius, J. (1995) Psychoanalytic understanding and nursing: A supervisory workshop with nurse tutors. *Psychoanalytic Psychotherapy* **9**: 17–29.

Figlio, K. (1987) The lost subject of sociology. In *Sociological Theory and Medical Sociology*, Scambler, G. (editor), London: Tavistock Publications 77–109.

Fineman, S. (1993) (editor) *Emotions in Organisations*. London: Sage.

Fineman, S. (2004) Getting the measure of emotion – and the cautionary tale of emotional intelligence. *Human Relations* **57**(6): 719–740.

Foucault, M. (1979) *Discipline and Punish: The birth of the prison*. New York: Vintage.

Forrest, D. (1989) The experience of caring. *Journal of Advanced Nursing* **14**: 815–823.

Forss, A., Tishelman. C., Widmark, C. & Sachs, L. (2004) Women's experiences of cervical cellular changes: An unintentional transition from health to liminality? *Sociology of Health and Illness* **26**: 306–325.

Frank, D.I. (1989) Treatment preferences of infertile couples, *Applied Nursing Research* **2**(2): 94.

Franklin, S. (1990) Deconstructing desperateness: the social construction of infertility in popular representations of new reproductive technologies. In McNeil, M., Varcoe, I. & Yearley, S. (editors) *The New Reproductive Technologies*, Basingstoke: Macmillan 200–229.

Franklin, S. (1997) *Embodied Progress: A cultural account of assisted conception*. London: Routledge.

Freud, S. (1964) *Three Essays on the Theory of Sexuality, vol. VII, Complete Works of Sigmund Freud*. London: Hogarth Press/IPA.

Froggart, K. (1998) The place of metaphor and language in exploring nurses' emotional work. *Journal of Advanced Nursing.* **28**(2): 332–338.

Frost, P.J. (2003) *Toxic Emotions at Work*. Harvard: Harvard Business School Press.

Gadow, S. (1985) Nurse and patient: the caring relationship. In Bishop, A.H. & Scudder, J.R. (editors) *Caring, Curing, Coping, Nurse Physician, Patient Relationships*, Alabama: University of Alabama 31–43.

Gamarnikov, E. (1978) Sexual division of labour: the case of nursing In Kuhn, A. & Wolpe, A-M. (editors) *Feminism and Materialism*, London: Routledge and Kegan Paul.

Gardner, K.G. & Wheeler, E.C. (1981) Nurses' perceptions of the meaning of support in nursing. *Issues in Mental Health Nursing* **3**: 13–28.

Gardner, K.G. & Wheeler, E.C. (1987) Patients' perceptions of support. *Western Journal of Nursing Research* **9**: 115–131.

Managing intimacy and emotions

Gerth, H. & Wright-Mills, C. (1964) *Character and Social Structure: The Psychology of Social Institutions*, New York: Harcourt, Brace and World.

Gilligan, C. (1982) in *A Different Voice: psychological theory and women's development*. Cambridge, Massachusetts: Harvard University Press.

Gilligan, C. (1993) *In A Different Voice: psychological theory and women's development*, 2nd edn. London: Harvard University Press.

Girard, M. (1988) Technical expertise as an ethical form: towards an ethics of distance. *Journal of Medical Ethics* 14: 25–30.

Glover, L., Hunter, M., Richards, J.M., Katz, M. & Abel P.D. (1999) Development of the fertility adjustment scale. *Fertility & Sterility* **72**(4): 623–628.

Goffman, I. (1959) *The Presentation of Self in Everyday Life*. London: Penguin Books.

Golombok, S., Cook, R., Bish, A. & Murray, C. (1993) Quality of parenting in families created by the new reproductive technologies: a brief report of preliminary findings. *Journal of Psychosomatic Obstetrics and Gynaecology* **14**: 17–22.

Golombok, S., Cook, R., Bish, A., & Murray, C. (1995) Families created by the new reproductive technologies: quality of parenting and social and emotional development of the children. *Child Development* **66**(22): 285–298.

Golombok, S., Brewaeys, A., Cook, R., Giavazzi, M.T., Guerra, D., Mantovani, A., van Hall, E., Crosignani, P.G., & Dexeus, S. (1996) Children: The European study of assisted reproduction families: family functioning and child development. *Human Reproduction* **11**(10): 2324–2331.

Gomm, R., Hammersley, M. & Foster, P. (2000) (editors). *Case Study Method*. London: SAGE.

Gorovitz, S. (1994) Is caring a viable component of health care? *Health Care Analysis* **2**(2): 129–133.

Graham, H. (1993) Social divisions in caring. *Women's Studies International Forum* **16**(5): 461–470.

Greenfield, D. and Haseltine, F. (1986) Candidate selection and psychosocial considerations of in-vitro fertilisation procedures. *Clinical Obstetrics and Gynecology* **29**(1): 119–125.

Greer, G. (2005) Afterword. In *Inconceivable Conceptions: Psychological aspects of infertility and reproductive technology*, Haynes, J. and Miller, J. (editors) (afterword by Germaine Greer). Hove and New York: Brunner-Routledge 207–216..

Greil, A.L. (1991) A secret stigma: The analogy between infertility and chronic illness and disability. In *Advances in Medical Sociology*, vol. 2, Albrecht, G.L. & Levy, J.A. (editors). Boston: JAI Press Inc. 49–62

Greil, A.L. (1997) Infertility and psychological distress: A critical review of the literature. *Social Science & Medicine* **45**(11): 1679–1704.

Griffiths, P., Barnes, E. & Ord, J. (1998) *Face to Face with Distress: the Professional Use of Self in Psychosocial Care*. London: Elsevier Health Sciences.

Griffin, A.P. (1983) A philosophical analysis of caring. *Journal of Advanced Nursing* **8**(4): 289–295.

Grosz, E. (1994) *Volatile Bodies: Towards a corporeal feminism*. Bloomington, IN: Indiana University Press.

Halldorsdottir, S. & Hamrin, E. (1997) Caring and uncaring encounters within nursing and health care from the cancer patient's perspective. *Cancer Nursing*, April: 120–128.

Halman, L.J., Andrews, F.M. & Abbey, A. (1994) Gender differences and perceptions about childbearing among infertile couples. *Journal of Obstetric, Gynecologic and Neonatal Nursing*, **23**(7): 593–600.

Haraway, D. (1992) The biopolitics of postmodern bodies: determinations of self in immune system discourse. *Differences: A Journal of Feminist Cultural Studies* **1**: 3–43.

Harbison, J. (1992) Gilligan: a voice for nursing? *Journal of Medical Ethics* **18**(4): 202–205.

Hartman, P. (1998) Revisiting the call to care: an ethical perspective. *Advances in Nursing Practice Quarterly* **4**(2): 14–18.

Hartigan, P. (2001) The importance of gender in defining and improving quality of care: some conceptual issues. *Health Policy and Planning* **16**(Suppl.1): 7–12.

Hawthorne, D.L. & Yurkovich, N.J. (1995) Science, technology, caring and the professions: are they compatible? *Journal of Advanced Nursing* **21**(6): 1087–1091.

Heagerty, B.V. (1990) *Class, Gender and Professionalisation: The struggle for British midwifery: 1900–1936.* Michigan: Department of History, Michigan State University.

Hearn, J. (1982) Notes on patriarchy, professionalisation and the semi-professions. *Sociology* **16**(2): 184–202.

Hjelmstedt, A. (2003). Patterns of emotional responses to pregnancy, experience of pregnancy and attitudes to parenthood among IVF couples: a longitudinal study. *Journal of Psychosomatic Obstetrics & Gynaecology*, **24**: 15 –162.

Hjelmstedt, A., Widstrom, A.M., Wramsby, H., & Collins, A. (2004). Emotional adaptation following successful in vitro fertilisation. *Fertility & Sterility* **81**: 1254–1264.

Heslop, L. & Oates, J. (1995) The discursive formation of caring. In Gray, G. and Pratt, R. (editors) *Scholarship in the Discipline of Nursing*, Melbourne Australia: Churchill Livingstone 255–276.

Hinks, J.A., Jenkins, J. & Corrigan, E. (2002) *Survey of the Continuity of Nursing Care in UK IVF Clinics.* Abstracts of the 18th Annual Meeting of the ESHRE Vienna, Austria 2002.

Hirsch, A.M. & Hirsch, S.M. (1989) The effect of infertility on marriage and self-concept, *Journal of Obstetric, Gynecologic and Neonatal Nursing* **18**(1): 13–20.

Hochschild, A.R. (1983) *The Managed Heart: commercialisation of human feeling.* Berkeley, CA: University of California Press.

Hochschild, A. (1995) The culture of politics: traditional, postmodern, cold-modern, and warm-modern ideals of care. *Social Politics* **2**(3) 331–346.

Horney, K. (1967) *Feminine Psychology* New York: Norton.

Horrocks, S., Anderson, E. & Salisbury, C. (2002) Systematic review of whether nurse practitioners working in primary care can provide equivalent care to doctors. *British Medical Journal* **324**: 819–823.

Howell-White, S. (1999) Choosing a birth attendant: The influences of a women's childbirth definition. *Social Science and Medicine* **45**: 925–36.

Hughes, E.C., Hughes, H.M. & Deutscher, I. (1958) *Twenty Thousand Nurses Tell their Story.* Philadelphia: J B Lippincott Co.

Hugman, R. (1998) *Social Welfare and Social Value: the role of caring professions.* Oxford: Macmillan.

Hull, M.R.G. (1992) Expectations of assisted conception for infertility. *British Medical Journal* **304**, June 6: 1465–1469.

Human Fertilisation and Embryology Authority (2000) *Ninth Annual Report & Accounts.* London: HFEA.

Human Fertilisation and Embryology Authority (2005/2006) Annual Statistics. http://www.hfea.gov.uk/en/406.html. (Accessed 31/07/08).

Human Fertilisation and Embryology Authority (2008) HFEA Long Term Register Data Analysis. http://www.hfea.gov.uk/en/1540.html#latest_edition. (Accessed 31/07/08).

Hunt, J.C. (1989) *Psychoanalytic Aspects of Fieldwork*, Qualitative Research Methods Series, 18, London: Sage Publications.

Hunt, M. & Meerabeau, L. (1993) Purging the emotions: the lack of emotional expression in subfertility and in the care of the dying. *International Journal of Nursing Studies* **30**(2): 115–123.

Hunt, J. & Monach, J. (1997) Beyond the bereavement model – the significance of depression for infertility counselling. *Human Reproduction, Supplement, Journal of British Fertility Society* **2**(2): 188–194.

Irwin, R. (2002) *Psychosexual Nursing.* London: Whurr Publishers Ltd.

Irwin, R. (2006) Thirty years of psychosexual nursing. *Sexual and Relationship Therapy* **21**(4): 445–461.

Jackson, S. (1993) Even sociologists fall in love: an exploration in the sociology of emotions. *Sociology* **27**: 201–220.

James, N. (1992) Care = Organisation + Physical Labour + Emotional Labour. *Sociology of Health and Illness* **14**(4): 488–507.

James, W. & Lange, C.G. (1922) *The Emotions*. Baltimore, MD: Williams and Wilkins.

Jones, S.L. (1994) Assisted reproductive technologies: genetic and nursing implications. *Journal of Obstetric, Gynecologic and Neonatal Nursing* **23**(6): 492–497.

Jones, L. & Webb, C. (1994) Young men's experiences of testicular cancer. In *Living Sexuality: Issues for nursing and health*, Webb, C. (editor) London: Scutari Press 32–49.

Katz, R.S. (2006) *When Professionals Weep: emotional and countertransference responses in end-of-life care*. London: Routledge.

Kitson, A.L. (1987) A comparative analysis of lay-caring and professional (nursing) caring relationships. *International Journal of Nursing Studies* **24**(2): 155–165.

Kitson, A. (1999) The essence of nursing. *Nursing Standard* **24**(13): 42–6.

Kirschenbaum, H. & Henderson, V.L. (editors) (1989) *Rogers Carl: Dialogues, Conversations with Martin Buber, Paul Tillich, B F Skinner, Gregory Bateson, Michael Polyani, Rollo May and others*. Boston: Houghton Mifflin Co.

Klein, M. (1975) *Envy and Gratitude and Other Works 1946–1963*. London: The Hogarth Trust.

Koropatrick, S. (1993) Infertility: A non-event transition. *Fertility and Sterility* **59**(1): 163–171.

Kübler-Ross, E. (1973) *On Death and Dying*, London: Tavistock/Routledge.

Kuhse, H. (1997) *Caring: Nurses, women and ethics*. Oxford: Blackwell.

Kyle, T.V. (1995) The concept of caring. *Journal of Advanced Nursing* **21**(3): 506–514.

Land, L., Ni Mhaolrúnaigh, S. & Castledine, G. (1996) Extent and effectiveness of the scope of professional practice. *Nursing Times* **92**(35): 32–35.

Lawler, J. (1990) *Behind the Screens: Nursing, somology and the problem of the body*. London: Churchill Livingstone.

Lay, M.M. (2000) *The Rhetoric of Midwifery: Gender, knowledge and power*. New Brunsick, MN: Rutgers University Press.

Leiblum, S.R., Aviv, A., & Hamer, R. (1998). Life after infertility: a long-term investigation of marital and sexual function. *Human Reproduction* **13**: 3569–3574.

Leininger, M. (1978) *Transcultural Caring – Concepts, Theories and Practices*. New York: Wiley.

Leininger, M. (1990) Historic and epistemologic dimensions of care and caring with future dimensions. In Stevenson, J.S. & Tripp-Reimer, T. (editors) *Knowledge about Care and Caring: the State of Art and Future Developments*. New York: American Academy of Nursing 19–31.

Lincoln, Y. & Guba, E. G. (2000) The only generalisation is: there is no generalisation. In Gomm, R, & Hammersley, M. and Foster, P. (editors) *Case Study Method* London: Sage Publications Ltd. 27–44.

Luker, K.A. (1997) Research and the configuration of nursing services. *Journal of Clinical Nursing* **6**: 259–267.

Lupton, D. (1995) Perspectives on power, communication and the medical encounter: implications for nursing theory and practice. *Nursing Inquiry* **2**(3): 157–163.

MacDonald, J.J. (1993) *Primary Health Care: Medicine in its place*. London: EarthScan Publications Ltd.

McCormick, T.M. (1980) Out of control: one aspect of infertility. *Journal of Obstetrics, Gynecology and Neonatal Nursing* **9**(3): 205–206.

McKenna, H. (1995) Nursing skill mix substitution and quality of care: an exploration of assumptions from the research and literature. *Journal of Advanced Nursing* **2**(3): 452–459.

McMahon, C.A., Gibson, F., Leslie, G., Cohen, J., & Tennant, C. (2003). Parents of in vitro fertilisation children: psychological adjustment, parenting, stress and the influence of subsequent in vitro fertilisation treatment. *Journal of Family Psychology* **17**: 361–369.

Mahlstedt, P.P. (1991) What is essential is invisible to the eye: dealing with patient disappointment. In Garner, C. (editor) *Principles of Infertility Nursing*. Boca Raton, FL: CRC Press, 157–167.

Main, T. (1968) The ailment. In Barnes, E. (editor) *Psychosocial Nursing: Studies from the Cassell Hospital* London: Tavistock Publications 12–35.

Malin, M., Hemmicki, E., Raikkonen, O., Sihvo, S., & Perala, M.-L. (2001). What do women want? Women's experiences of infertility treatment. *Social Science & Medicine* **53**: 123–331.

Manley, K. (1997) Operationalising an advanced practice/consultant nurse role: an action research study. *Journal of Clinical Nursing* **6**(3): 179–190.

Manley, K. & Garbett, R. (2000) Paying Peter and Paul: reconciling concepts of expertise with competency for a clinical career structure. *Journal of Clinical Nursing* **9**(3): 347–359.

Martin, E. (1987) *The Woman in the Body: A cultural analysis of reproduction*. Boston: Beacon Press.

Matthews, R. & Matthews, A.M. (1986) Infertility and involuntary childlessness. *Journal of Marriage and the Family* **48**(8): 641–649.

May, C. (1990) Research on nurse-patient relationships: problems of theory, problems of practice. *Journal of Advanced Nursing* **15**(3): 307–315.

May, C. (1991) Affective neutrality and involvement in nurse/patient relationships: perceptions of appropriate behaviours among nurses in acute medical and surgical wards. *Journal of Advanced Nursing* **16**: 552–58.

Meerabeau, L. (1999) The management of embarrassment and sexuality in health care. *Journal of Advanced Nursing* **29**: 1507–1513.

Meerabeau, L. & Denton, J. eds. (1995) *Infertility Nursing and Caring*. London: Scutari Press.

Menning, B.E. (1977) *Infertility, a guide for childless couples* New Jersey: Prentice-Hall Inc.

Menning, B.E. (1980) The emotional needs of infertile couples. *Fertility and Sterility* **34**(4): 313–319.

Menzies, I.E.P. (1970) *The Functioning of Social Systems as a Defence against Anxiety*. London: The Tavistock Institute of Human Relations.

Merleau-Ponty, M. (1962) *Phenomenology of Perception*. London: Routledge and Kegan Paul.

Meutzal, A.P. (1988) Therapeutic nursing. In Pearson, A. (editor). *Primary Nursing: nursing in the Burford and Oxford nursing development units*. London: Chapman and Hall 89–116.

Miers, M. (2000) Gender issues and nursing practice. Macmillan: Basingstoke.

Millard, S. (1991) Emotional responses to infertility, *Association of Peri-operative Registered Nurses Journal*, **54**(2): 301–305.

Miller, J. (2005) Mourning the never born and the loss of the angel. In Haynes, J. & Miller, J. (editors) *Inconceivable Conceptions: Psychological aspects of infertility and reproductive technology* (afterword by Germaine Greer). Hove and New York: Brunner-Routledge 47–59.

Milne, B.J. (1988) Couples' experiences with in vitro fertilisation. *Journal of Obstetric, Gynecologic and Neonatal Nursing* **17**(5): 347–352.

Mitchell, J. (1974) *Psychoanalysis and Feminism*. Harmondsworth: Pelican.

Morse, J. (1991) Negotiating commitment and involvement in the nurse-patient relationship. *Journal of Advanced Nursing* **16**(4): 455–468.

Morse, J.M., Solberg, S.M., Neander, W.L. & Bottorff, J.L. (1990) Concepts of caring and caring as a concept. *Advances in Nursing Science* **13**(1): 1–14.

Managing intimacy and emotions

Morse, J., Andeson, G., Bottoroff, J.L., Yonge, O., O'Brien, B., Solberg, S.M. & McIlveen, H. (1992) Exploring Empathy: a conceptual fit for nursing? *IMAGE: Journal of Nursing Scholarship* **24**(4): 273–280.

MRC Working Party on Children Conceived by IVF (1990) Births in Great Britain resulting from assisted conception. *British Medical Journal* **300**: 1229–1233.

Muff, J. (1982) *Socialisation, Sexism and Stereotyping Women's Issues*, St Louis: C V Mosby.

Murray Parkes, C. (1998) Facing loss. *British Medical Journal* **316**:1521–1524.

Nightingale, F. (1859) *Notes on Nursing, What it is and what it is not*. London: Harrison, reprint (1980) New York: Churchill Livingstone.

Noddings, N. (1984) *Caring: A Feminine Approach to Ethics and Moral Education*. Berkeley: University of California Press.

Oakley, A. (1993) *Essays on Women, Medicine and Health*, Edinburgh: Edinburgh University Press.

Obholzer, A. (1993) Institutional forces. *Therapeutic Communities* **14**(4): 275–282.

Obholzer, A. (2003) Managing social anxieties in public sector organisations. In Reynolds, J. (editor) *Managing Care Reader*. London: Routledge.

Obholzer, A. & Zagier Roberts, V. (1994) *The Unconscious at Work, Individual and Organisational Stress in the Human Services*. London: Routledge.

Olshansky, E.F. (1987) Identity of self as infertile: An example of theory-generating research. *Advances in Nursing Science* **9**: 54–63.

Orbach, S. (1999) Listening to your analyst. *LSE Magazine* **11**(1): 12–13.

Paley, J. (2001) An archaeology of caring knowledge. *Journal of Advanced Nursing* **36**(2): 188–198.

Pellegrino, E.D. (1983) The caring ethic: the relation of physician to patient. In Bishop, A.H. & Scudder, J.R. (editors) *Caring, Curing, Coping: nurse physician, patient relationships*. Alabama: University of Alabama 8–30.

Peplau, H. (1969) Professional closeness. *Nursing Forum* **8**(4): 342–360.

Peplau, H. (1988) *Interpersonal Relations in Nursing*. London: Macmillan Education Ltd.

Pfeffer, N. (1993) *The Stork and the Syringe. A political history of reproductive medicine*. Cambridge: Polity Press.

Phillips, D.Z. (1983) Can you become a professional friend? *The Gadlfy* **5**: 29–43.

Phillips, S. (1996) Labouring the emotions: expanding the remit of nursing work? *Journal of Advanced Nursing* **24**(1): 139–143.

Pietroni, P. (1993) Attachment and non-attachment. *Journal of Psychoanalytic Psychology* **38**(1): 45–55.

Pines, D. (1993) *A Woman's Unconscious Use of her Body*. London: Virago.

Porter, M. (1990) Professional–client relationships and women's reproductive healthcare. In Cunningham-Burley, S. & McKeganey, N.P. (editors) *Readings in Medical Sociology*. New York: Tavistock Routledge 182–254.

Porter, S. (1992) Women in a women's job: the gendered experience of nurses. *Journal of Advanced Nursing* **14**(4): 510–527.

Porter, S. (1995) *Nursing's Relationship with Medicine*. Aldershot: Avebury.

Porter, S. (1998) *Social Theory and Nursing Practice*. London: Macmillan Press Ltd.

Prattke, T.W. & Gass-Sternas, K.A. (1993) Appraisal, coping and emotional health of infertile couples undergoing donor artificial insemination. *Journal of Obstetric, Gynecologic and Neonatal Nursing* **22**(6): 516–527.

Price, J. & Schildrick, M. (editors) (1999) *Feminist Theory and the Body, a reader*. Edinburgh: Edinburgh University Press.

Purkiss, M.E. (1996) Nursing in quality space: technologies governing experiences of care. *Nursing Inquiry* **3**(2): 101–111.

Qureshi, H. & Walker, A. (1990) *The Caring Relationship: elderly people and their families*. Basingstoke: Macmillan Education Ltd.

Qureshi, N.S., Walker, S.E., Pike, D.J. & Murray, A. (1997) Transport in vitro fertilisation: three years experience at a general district hospital. *Journal of Obstetrics & Gynaecology.* **17**(5): 457–460.

Raphael-Leff, J. (1991) *Psychological Processes of Childbearing*. London: Chapman & Hall.

Ray, M.A. (1987) Technological caring: a new model in critical care. *Dimensions of Critical Care* **6**: 166–173.

Reiman, D. (1986) Non-caring and caring in the clinical setting. *Topics of Clinical Nursing* **2**(1): 30–36.

Reverby, S. (1987) A caring dilemma: Womanhood and nursing in historical perspective. *Nursing Research* **36**: 5–11.

Robertson, D. & Freshwater, D. (2002) *Emotions and Needs*. Buckingham: Open University Press.

Rogers, C. (1951) *The Application of Client Centred Therapy*. London: Constable.

Rogers, C. (1975) *The Counselling Psychologist*. London: Constable.

Rogers, C. (1967) *On Becoming a Person, A therapist's view of psychotherapy*. London: Constable.

Rose, G. (1993) *Feminism and Geography: the limits of geographical knowledge*. Cambridge: Polity Press; Minneapolis, MN: University of Minnesota Press.

Ross, M.R.H.C. (1995) The gynaecology unit – a psychodynamic perspective. *Psychodynamic Counselling* **1**(2): 199–211.

Rossen, E.K. & Gruber, K.J. (2007) Development and testing of the relocation self-efficacy scale. *Nursing Research* **56**(4): 244–251.

Royal College of Obstetricians and Gynaecologists (1997) *Intimate Examinations: Report of a working party*. London: Royal College of Obstetricians and Gynaecologists.

Royal College of Nursing (2003) *The Future Nurse, a discussion paper*. London: RCN.

Royal College of Nursing (2007) *The Future Nurse: the RCN vision*. London: RCN.

Rudge, T. (1996) (Re)writing ethnography: The unsettling questions for nursing research raised by post-structural approaches to the field. *Nursing Inquiry* **3**: 146–52.

Salvage, J. (1990) The theory and practice of the 'new nursing'. *Nursing Times* **86**(4): 42–45.

Salvage, J. & Heijnen, S. (1997) Nursing and midwifery in Europe. In Salvage, J. & Heijnen, S. (editors) *Nursing in Europe a resource for better health*. WHO Regional Publications, European Series (number 74): 21–126.

Sanford, R.C. (2000) Caring through relation and dialogue :a nursing perspective for patient education. *Advances in Nursing Science* **22**(3): 1–15.

Sandelowski, M. (1990) Failures of volition: female agency and infertility in historical perspective. *Signs* **15**(3): 475–499.

Sandelowski, M. (1993) *With Child in Mind. Studies of the personal encounter with infertility*. Philadelphia: University of Pennsylvania Press.

Sandelowski, M. (1995) A theory of transition to parenthood of infertile couples. *Research in Nursing and Health* **18**: 123–32.

Sandelowski, M., Holditch-Davis, D. & Harris, B.G. (1990) Living the life: Explanations of infertility. *Sociology of Health and Illness* **12**: 195–215.

Savage, J. (1995) *Nursing Intimacy*. London: Scutari Press.

Savage, J. (2003) *Emotional Work and Balint. Emotions in practice. A study of Balint seminar training as experiential learning for qualified nurses*. London: Royal College of Nursing.

Sayers, J. (1991) *Mothering Psychoanalysis*. London: Hamish Hamilton.

Schildrick, M. (1997) *Leaky Bodies and Boundaries: Feminism, postmodernism and (bio)ethics*. London: Routledge.

Managing intimacy and emotions

Schilling, C. (2003) *The Body and Social Theory*, 2nd edn. London: Sage Publications.

Schmidt, L., Holstein, B.E., Christensen, U. & Boivin, J. (2005) Communication and coping as predictors of fertility problem stress: cohort study of 186 participants who did not achieve a delivery after 12 months of fertility treatment. *Human Reproduction* **20**(11): 3248–3256.

Selby, J. (1990) Psychosexual nursing. In Skrine, R. (editor) *Introduction to Psychosexual medicine*. London: Chapman and Hall 134–147.

Smith, P. (1992) *The Emotional Labour of Nursing; how nurses care*. Basingstoke: Macmillan.

Smith, P. & Agard, E. (1997) Care costs: towards a critical understanding of care. In Brykczynska, G. (editor) *Caring: the compassion and wisdom of nursing*. London: Arnold 180–204.

Souter, V.L. (1997) A survey of infertility practices in Scotland. *British Journal of General Practice* **47**(424): 727–728.

Spiers, J.A. (1998) The use of face work and politeness theory, *Qualitative Health Research* **8**(1): 25–47.

Spilsbury, K. & Meyer, J. (2001) Defining the nursing contribution to patient outcome: lessons from a review of the literature examining nursing outcomes, skill mix and changing roles. *Journal of Clinical Nursing* **10**: 3–14.

Strang, J. (1982) Psychotherapy by nurses - some special characteristics. *Journal of Advanced Nursing* **7**: 167–171.

Strauss, A., Fagerhaugh, S., Suczek, B. and Wiener, C. (1982) Sentimental work in the technologised hospital. *Sociology of Health and Illness* **4**(3): 254–278.

Street, A.F. (1992) *Inside Nursing: a critical ethnography of clinical nursing practice*. New York: State University of New York.

Swanson, K.M. (1999) Effects of caring, measurement, and time on miscarriage impact on women's well-being. *Nursing Research* **48**(6): 288–298.

Synott, A. (1993) *The Body Social, Symbolism, Self and Society*. London: Routledge.

Taylor, D. (personal communication) *What immortal hand or eye has framed thy fearful symmetry?*

Temmink, D., Francke, A.L., Hutten, J.B.F., van der Zee, J. & Ahuijer Abu-Said, H. (2000) Innovations in the nursing care of the chronically ill: a literature review from an international perspective. *Journal of Advanced Nursing* **31**(6): 1449–1458.

Thomas, C. (1993) Deconstructing concepts of care. *Sociology* **27**(4): 649–669.

Thomas, L.H. (1994) A comparison of the verbal interactions of qualified nurses and nursing auxilliaries in primary, team and functional nursing wards. *International Journal of Nursing Studies* **31**(3): 231–244.

Tjørnhøj-Thomsen, T. (2005) Close encounters with infertility and procreative technology. In *Managing uncertainty. Ethnographic studies of illness, risk and the struggle for control*, Steffen, M., Jenkins, R., & Jessen, H. (editors) Copenhagen: Museum Tusculnum Press, University of Copenhagen 21–92.

Tong, R. (1994) *Feminist Thought: a comprehensive introduction*. London: Routledge.

Torrance, C.J., Das, R. & Allison, C.M. (1999) Use of chaperones in clinics for genitourinary medicine: Survey of consultants. *British Medical Journal* **319**: 159–60.

Travelbee, J. (1971) *Interpersonal Aspects of Nursing* (2nd Edition). Philadelphia: FA Davies.

Tubert, S. (2004) *Women without a Shadow. Maternal desire and assisted reproductive technologies*. London: Free Association Books.

Turner, J.H. (2007) *Human Emotions: a sociological theory*. London: Routledge.

Tutton, E. (1991) An exploration of touch and its use in nursing. In McMahon, R., Pearson, A. (editors). *Nursing as therapy*. London: Chapman & Hall, 142–169.

UKCC (1992) *The Scope of Professional Practice*. London: UKCC.

UKCC (1996) *The Nature of Advanced Practice: an Interim Report* London: UKCC.

UKCC (1997) *Scope in Practice*. London: UKCC.

UKCC (1998) *The Future of Professional Regulation*. London: UKCC.

UKCC (1999a) *A Higher Level of Practice - Pilot Standard*. London: UKCC.

UKCC (1999b) *Healthcare Futures 2010*. London: UKCC.

UKCC (1999c) *Fitness for Practice*. London: UKCC.

UKCC (2002) *Report of the Higher Level of Practice Pilot and Project - Executive summary*. London: UKCC.

Uys, L.R. (1980) Towards the development of an operational definition of the concept 'therapeutic use of self'. *Journal Nursing Studies* **17**: 175–180.

van Dongen, E. & Elema, R. (2001) The art of touching: the culture of 'body work' in nursing. *Anthropology and Medicine* **8**(2/3): 149–162.

Van Essen, L. & Sjoden, P. (1991) Patients and staff's perceptions of caring: a review and replication, *Journal of Advanced Nursing* **16**(11): 1363–1374.

Van Gennep, A. (1960/1909) *Rites of passage. (Les rites de passage)* (translated by MB Vizedom and GL Caffee). Chicago: The University of Chicago Press.

Van Shie, T. & Seedhouse, D. (1997) The importance of care. *Health Care Analysis*. **5**(4): 283–291.

Wallach, E.E. (1980) The frustrations of being 'normal' yet infertile. *Fertility and Sterility* **34**: 405–406.

Walter, L. (1995) Feminist anthropology? *Gender and Society* **9**: 272–288.

Warner, J. & Gabe, J. (2004) Risk and liminality in mental health social work. *Health, Risk and Society* **6**: 387–399.

Warr, J. (1998) An evaluative study into the effectiveness of level 3 national vocational qualification support staff to nurses. *Nurse Education Today* **18**(6): 505–516.

Waterworth, S. & Luker, K.A. (1990) Reluctant collaborators: do patients want to be involved in decisions concerning care, *Journal of Advanced Nursing* **15**(8): 971–976.

Watson, J. (1988) *Nursing: human science and human caring - a theory of nursing*. New York: National League for Nursing.

Weaver, S.M., Clifford, E., Gordon, A.G., Hay, A.M., & Robinson, J. (1993). A follow-up study of 'successful' IVF/ GIFT couples: social - emotional well being and adjustment to parenthood. *Journal of Psychosomatic Obstetrics & Gynaecology* **14** (Suppl.), 5–16.

Weedon, C. (1997) *Feminist Practice and Poststructuralist Theory* (2nd Edition). Oxford: Blackwell Publishers Inc.

Wells, D. (2000) *Caring for Sexuality in Health and Illness*. Churchill Livingstone.

Whittaker, D. (1993) *In the Room - invisible work and hidden experiences of women nurses and women patients in a GUM clinic*. MSc Thesis, University of London.

Williams, A. (1990) Reflections on the making of an ethnographic text. *Studies in Sexual Politics* no. 29. Manchester: Manchester University Press.

Williams, A. (2000) *Nursing, Medicine and Primary Care*. Buckingham: Open University Press.

Williams, A. (2001) A study of practising nurses' perceptions and experiences of intimacy within the nurse-patient relationship. *Journal of Advanced Nursing* **35**(2): 188–196.

Williams, S. (1997) Modern medicine and the 'uncertain body': From corporeality to hyperreality? *Social Science and Medicine* **45**: 1041–1049.

Woods. L.P. (2000) *The Enigma of Advanced Nursing Practice*. Dinton, Wiltshire: Quay Books, Mark Allen Publishing Ltd.

Young, I.M. (1984) Pregnant embodiment: subjectivity and alienation. *Journal of Medicine and Philosophy* **9**: 45–62.

Managing intimacy and emotions

Websites:

www.dcnetwork.org (Accessed 27.02.09)

www.infertilitynetworkuk.com/moretolife/ (Accessed 09.02.09)

www.nice.org.uk/Guidance/CG11 (Accessed 27.02.09)

Index